Chinese Medicine for Aging Eyes

Hoy Ping Yee Chan, O.M.D.
Carole Conlon, L.Ac.

AyniWrite Press
ALBUQUERQUE NM

Copyright © 2014 by Authors Hoy Ping Yee Chan and Carole Conlon

All rights reserved. No part of this publication may be reproduced, distributed or transmitted in any form or by any means, including photocopying, recording, or other electronic or mechanical methods, without the prior written permission of the publisher, except in the case of brief quotations embodied in critical reviews and certain other noncommercial uses permitted by copyright law. For permission requests, write to the publisher, addressed "Attention: Permissions Coordinator," at the address below.

AyniWrite Press
10700 Academy Rd NE #2227 Albuquerque NM 87111
www.AyniWritePress.com

Book Layout ©2013 BookDesignTemplates.com

Chinese Medicine for Aging Eyes / Chan and Conlon —1st ed.
ISBN 978-0-9907550-0-5

Dedication

*This book was written in honor of
all dedicated
health care practitioners
and caregivers
serving
their senior eye patients,
addressing one of the leading
causes of disability in seniors
worldwide.*

"The eye is the lamp of the body.
If your eyes are good,
your whole body will be full of light.
But if your eyes are bad,
your whole body will be full of darkness."

(Matthew 6:22-23 a)

「眼睛就是身上的燈. 你的眼睛若瞭亮, 全身就光明;
你的眼睛若昏花, 全身就黑暗.」

(馬太福音 6:22-23 上)

Table of Contents

Dedication iii

Quote v

Preface xi

Acknowledgements xv

Introduction xvii

ONE
Traditional Chinese Medicine and Aging Eyes 1

TWO
Eye Examination 7

    1. Basic eye examination for Senior Patients 7
    2. Eye Observation Based on Western and Chinese Medicine 8
    3. Relative Terms of Normal Eye Anatomy and Physiological Functions ... 9
    4. Examination of the Palpebrae 13
    5. Examination of the Exterior Portion of the Anterior Eye 14

THREE
Blepharoptosis and Myasthenia 21

    1. Blepharoptosis 21
        o Causes of Blepharoptosis in Seniors 21
        o Examination 22
        o Symptoms 22
        o TCM Differential Diagnosis and Treatment 23
        o Prevention and Diet 26
    2. Myasthenia Gravis 27
        o Signs and Symptoms 27
        o TCM Differential Diagnosis and Treatment 28

FOUR
Dry Eye 31
    1. Causes of Dry Eye 31
    2. Symptoms 32
    3. TCM Differential Diagnosis and Treatment 32
    4. Formulas Used for External Treatment of Dry Eye 36
    5. Diet 39
    6. Prevention 40

FIVE
Glaucoma 43
    1. Causes of Glaucoma 43
    2. Forms of Glaucoma 44
    3. Risk Factors 44
    4. TCM Observation 44
    5. Primary Open-Angle Glaucoma 46
        ○ Symptoms 46
        ○ TCM Differential Diagnosis and Treatment 48
        ○ Prevention 51
        ○ Glaucoma Screening Exams 52
    6. Secondary Glaucoma 54

SIX
Senile Cataract 57
    1. Facts about Cataracts 57
    2. Cause and Prognosis 58
    3. Symptoms 59
    4. Learning from A Cataract Case 60
    5. TCM Differential Diagnosis and Treatment 61
    6. Dietary and Other Treatments 64
    7. Prevention 65

SEVEN
Vitreous Humor Diseases 69
    1. Floaters (Degeneration of the Vitreous) 69
    2. TCM Differential Diagnosis and Treatment 70
    3. Prevention 74

EIGHT
Age-Related Macular Degeneration **75**
    1. Facts About ARMD 75
    2. Risk Factors 76
    3. Symptoms 76
    4. The Structure and Pathophysiology of ARMD 79
    5. TCM Relationship Between the Macula and Organs 80
    6. TCM Differential Diagnosis and Treatment 82
    7. Common Western and Alternative Treatments for ARMD 87
    8. Prevention 88
    9. Chinese Herbal Diets 89

NINE
Retinopathy of Hypertension, Arteriosclerosis & Post-Stroke Dysopsia **95**
    1. Retinopathy of Hypertension and Arteriosclerosis 95
        ○   Factors Relating to These Diseases 95
        ○   Factors Relating to Secondary Hypertension 98
        ○   TCM Differential Diagnosis and Treatment 99
        ○   Ophthalmoscopic Changes Observed in Hypertension
            and Arteriosclerosis 102
        ○   Complications of Hypertension 104
        ○   Hypertensive Neuro-Retinopathy... 104
    2. Post-Stroke Dysopsia 106
        ○   Causes 106
        ○   Symptoms 106
        ○   Stroke Only Attacking the Eye 108
        ○   TCM Differential Diagnosis and Treatment 108
    3. Prevention of Hypertension, Arteriosclerosis and Stroke 109
        ○   General Rules for Stroke Prevention 109
        ○   Prevention Methods 110
    4. Transient Ischemic Attack (TIA) 111
        ○   The Seven Common TIA Symptoms 111
        ○   Self-Care Before the Occurrence of a Stroke 112

TEN
Retinopathy of Diabetes **117**
    1. Western Medical Symptoms and Diagnosis 117

    2. TCM Differential Diagnosis and Treatment 119
    3. Diet 123
    4. Prevention 124

ELEVEN
Occlusion **127**
    1. Central Retinal Artery Occlusion (CRAO) 127
        o Causes of Arterial Occlusion According to Western Medicine 128
        o TCM Pathogenesis of CRAO 128
        o TCM Differential Diagnosis and Treatment 129
        o Prevention 132
        o Ophthalmoscopic Changes Seen in CRAO 132
        o Complications 133
        o Other Medical Exams to Help Clarify a Diagnosis of Occlusion 133
    2. Central Retinal Vein Occlusion (CRVO) 134
        o Causes and Pathological Changes of CRVO
           According to Western Medicine 134
        o TCM Differential Diagnosis and Treatment 135
        o Ophthalmoscopic Changes Seen in CRVO 137
        o Complications 138
        o Prevention 138

TWELVE
Presbyopia **141**
    1. Symptoms 141
    2. Western Medical Treatment 142
    3. TCM Differential Diagnosis and Treatment 142
    4. Diet 144
    5. Prevention 144

THIRTEEN
General Prevention for Aging Eyes **149**
    1. Prevention Methods for Eye Care 149
    2. General Preventive Self-Care Method for Senior Health 153

Appendices **159**

- ONE: Introduction to Ocular Diagnosis and Periocular Acupuncture 159
  - Finding the Ocuzone Locations 159
  - Eight Regions and 13 Ocuzones 161
  - The Thirteen Ocuzones 161
  - Triple Warmer Theory of Ocular Acupuncture 163
  - The Principle of Therapeutic Selection of Ocuzones 165
  - Periocular Needling Technique 165
  - Precautionary Measures 168
  - Effects, Indications and Contraindications 170
- TWO: The Most Commonly Used Chinese Herbal Formula and Its Extensive Formulas for Aging Eyes and Body 173
- THREE: Eye Exercise Reading Chart 177
- FOUR: Common Eye Tests 179

Poem of Longevity **180**

General Index **181**

Formula Index **197**

Differential Diagnosis Index **199**

Treatment Principles Index **200**

About the Authors **203**

Preface

After working with a team of acupuncturists and physicians to compile the book *Acupuncture for Stroke Rehabilitation* published by Blue Poppy Press in 2006, I dreamed of writing another book but could not continue at that time because of declining health. I had gone through treatments of acupuncture, herbs, chiropractic, surgery and, at last, just rested to let my body slowly recover. Then in 2011, I had recovered enough energy to reactivate my dream. I meticulously thought about what subject I should write that would benefit our profession and patients and would fulfill my dream.

From April to June in 2012 I was given an opportunity by Bastyr University to teach a continuing education seminar on "Chinese Medicine for Senior Common Eye Disease". My teachings and handouts for the attendees received highest evaluations. This class helped make up my mind to turn the handouts into the book I wanted to write.

I have seen and experienced the development and growth of acupuncture and Chinese herbal treatment in Washington State and America over the last thirty years. The American public ranged from curious to accepting of acupuncture and I watched acupuncture move from being illegal to legal; from patients paying out of pocket for treatment to now being covered by most medical and car insurance companies; from only being known as helpful for pain relief to being accepted for the treatment of other diseases. I was very happy to see the step by step acceptance for acupuncture in America by medical professionals and medical insurance companies. I have to clear the misunderstanding here in the United States where most people place acupuncture outside the context of traditional Chinese medicine. Actually, acupuncture is just one part of TCM. Unfortunately the acceptance of acupuncture does not mean traditional Chinese medicine has been fully accepted. The progression towards full acceptance of integrated traditional Chinese and Western medicine as a new healing method to benefit people is taking too long.

Among all the clinical healings, I think the eye is the hardest area to make this East-West integration in the United States. Many of my patients who have gone to see ophthalmologists were given very good eye exams and diagnoses but without appropriate treatments being offered. For this reason they turned to me, expecting some help for their eye conditions. Some doctors noticed that acupuncture and Chinese herbs gave good results but ignored them and explained to their patients that the vision improvements were only due to natural healing and ignored positive effects provided by any other practitioner.

However, there was one ophthalmologist specializing in glaucoma, who agreed his patient's intraocular pressure and optic nerve could be kept under control by combining prescribed eye drops with my acupuncture treatments. He encouraged this patient to continue what he was doing. Another optometrist referred many of his family members and patients to me because he recognized the good results they experienced. He often came into my office to take my brochures and pamphlets for display in his office. I extremely appreciated these two exceptional doctors for being so open-minded to the benefits of Chinese medicine.

Because of these experiences, I thought that a book in English, detailing how traditional Chinese medicine can help some difficult eye conditions, will hopefully shorten the time it takes for the creation of a new, integrated medical method to benefit eye patients. As an example, it is very common in China where many doctors work in eye clinics and hospitals using a combination of both Western and traditional Chinese medicine, to treat eye disease with good results. Even in the early 70's when I was in China working in the eye department of a hospital, we used this combined method to treat eye diseases.

There is another problem slowing down the integration of Western and TCM method for treating eye diseases - and that weakness is our own profession. I do not know how many acupuncture schools in the nation offer a full academic course to teach eye diseases; there may be a few or perhaps even none? I have taught many continuing education seminars in the United States and know from the attendees (licensed acupuncturists) that many of them do not know the anatomy of the eye or the Western diagnosis of eye diseases. I wonder how they can do well in their work and have good communication with their eye patients and doctors? I honestly encourage our young acupuncturists to learn TCM for treating eye conditions in depth and to acquire some Western medical knowledge of eye diseases. This will help if you want to obtain optimum beneficial results from your eye treatments, thus making your patients happy about your work. It will also benefit eye care health in this nation due to improved communication between practitioners of both treatment approaches and the wisdom of understanding both. Because of this, I have included basic

Western medical knowledge about the eye to help acupuncturists be more effective using TCM for treating eye diseases.

Although traditional Chinese medicine can treat many difficult eye conditions, it has weak points too which I will discuss in Chapter One of this book. I firmly believe that especially in the treatment of eye diseases, practitioners of both Western and traditional Chinese medicine should combine their unique expertise to complement each method's strengths and counter any weaknesses. Practitioners need to see that it is good to use a combination of both medicines to obtain best results. My hope is that a new, integrated method for treatment of the eyes will be developed soon in United States and will spread throughout the world.

Thank you very much for your interest in this book. Because of my limited knowledge, my health, and my age, I focused the subject to senior aging eyes because seniors have more eye diseases and, if these problems are not taken care of, may ultimately lead to blindness. After reading the contents of this book, you will understand how important it is to take care of the eyes of seniors, thus giving them comfortable and happy lives. It will benefit not only seniors and their families but also the economy and our society as a whole.

Please excuse any mistakes in this book.

I welcome any comments.

Hoy Ping Yee Chan, OMD
Diplomate of Acupuncture, Retired NCCAOM
Diplomate of Chinese Herbology, Retired NCCAOM
Everett, Washington, U.S.A.
June 2014

Acknowledgements

This book owes its successful completion to the following people who helped in different ways to support the writing and publishing.

Carole Conlon, L.Ac., my fledgling student who graduated in 1984 from the Northwest Institute of Acupuncture and Oriental Medicine. She is now my good friend. Carole has spent a lot of time and energy to turn my original class handout of "Chinese Medicine for Senior Common Eye Diseases" into this book. One of her areas of expertise is drawing and she drew most of the illustrations in this book. Without her strong support and excellent work, her honorable friendship, this book might not have been published.

Philina Chan, my granddaughter is a computer graphic designer. She used her day off during a Christmas visit to Seattle to make the cover of this book.

Dong H. Chan, my husband who supported my seminar teaching by volunteering to be my patient in order to demonstrate the periocular acupuncture techniques for the attendees. He also supported me in writing this book.

For the endless love of my other family members who supported me after we immigrated to the U.S., helping me dedicate more than 30 years of my life to the profession of traditional Chinese medicine. Their help gave me the chance to succeed in writing this book.

Special thank you goes to the publisher of AyniWrite Press for being willing to publish this book.

I also want to thank all acupuncturists who had referred eye patients to me during my twenty-five years clinical practice in the greater Seattle area. They gave me many chances to use acupuncture and Chinese herbal medicine and to explore the benefits in treating them. These referrals lead me to understand how important it was to push the integration of Western medicine and traditional Chinese medicine in the United States, and motivated me to write this book in my retirement.

Above all, I must give thanks to the faith that I believe in almighty God. Thank you. I thank Him for giving me health, energy and knowledge. Ultimately, it was by His wisdom, His grace, and His blessing that this work of love was accomplished.

Hoy Ping Yee Chan, O.M.D.

Introduction

Chinese Medicine for Aging Eyes joins the growing number of traditional Chinese medical books available to practitioners who are ready to increase their knowledge and skills in a specialty area - this one covering the treatment of eye diseases commonly seen in the senior patient. This book combines knowledge from both Eastern and Western medical approaches to help educate the acupuncturist and/or herbalist in diagnosis and treatment in a field where effective treatment is not easy or even always available! Ophthalmologists and optometrists can benefit from this book in order to understand the benefits traditional Chinese medicine can add to the successful treatment of eye diseases. Finally the senior eye patient can read about the disease that confronts them, learn about available treatment options for it in two medical systems, and adopt many methods of exercises, self-massage and supplementation that can help to slow or possibly stop eye disease progression.

The book discusses the strengths and weaknesses of both medical systems for the treatment of eye disease with the strong underlying message that a combined effort utilizing the strengths of each medical approach provides the best treatment for patients.

With this book, author Hoy Ping Yee Chan continues to build on the knowledge she presented in her 1996 book *Window of Health---Ocular Diagnosis and Periocular Acupuncture*.

In *Chinese Medicine for Aging Eyes* you will receive a brief introduction to the historical beginnings of eye healthcare in Chinese medicine as well as the correspondences between the eyes and the acupuncture meridians. There is also a brief review of the basics of eye anatomy and an introduction to the typical eye examinations done in the offices of ophthalmologists and optometrists. You will start to learn the special language those doctors use: O.D., O.U., O.S., LR, etc., and get a better understanding of the tools of their specialties. Ultimately this gives you, the practitioner, an improved ability to communicate more effectively with both your eye patient and his/her doctor, resulting in better care for the patient.

This book then gives an in-depth discussion of several of the most commonly seen eye diseases in the senior patient including blepharoptosis, myasthenia, dry eye, glaucoma, senile cataract, vitreous humor disease, macular degeneration, hypertension, arteriosclerosis, post-stroke dysopsia, TIA, diabetic retinopathy, occlusion, and presbyopia. These conditions are first presented in a Western medical context showing cause, diagnosis and treatment, followed by the traditional Chinese medical differential diagnosis and various treatment protocols using herbal formulas, filiform needles, tapping, scalp and ear needles as well as special periocular needling protocols using the ocuzones identified by Dr. Peng Jingshan.

Although *Chinese Medicine for Aging Eyes* is primarily written for the practitioner of Chinese medicine, the book contains an entire chapter dedicated to general health, diet and self-care methods for preventing or slowing the progress of eye disease. This information is valuable for a person especially interested in eye healthcare and can be used to better understand an eye condition he/she might be experiencing. This book clearly identifies the warning signs that these eye diseases give and shows ways to slow down or even stop their progression through exercises, supplements, and other methods.

The appendices of this book contain some very important excerpts from the book *Window of Health---Ocular Diagnosis and Periocular Acupuncture* that an acupuncturist must know before attempting needling near the eyes and surrounding blood vessels. It is recommended that anyone planning to use this needling technique purchase a copy of the complete book at www.Amazon.com (or the third edition is also available at http://www.lulu.com/content/1385515). The appendix also includes information on common eye tests, eye exercise charts, and the most common Chinese herbal formula and its many variations used for aging eyes.

Carole Conlon, L.Ac.
Diplomate of Acupuncture, NCCAOM
Albuquerque, NM U.S.A.
June 2014

CHAPTER ONE

Traditional Chinese Medicine and Aging Eyes

Traditional Chinese medicine has more than 4000 years history. The most famous book from this system of medicine is the *Huangdi Nei Jing*, the oldest and greatest medical classic. Its authorship is ascribed to the Ancient Emperor Huangdi (2698-2589 B.C.) but, in reality, the work was a product of various unknown authors in the Warring States Period (475-221 B.C.). The book consists of two parts: *Su Wen* (*Plain Questions*) and *Ling Shu* (*Miraculous Pivot*).

Both parts of the *Nei Jing* contain references to eye health. It was written in *Su Wen*: "All channels converge at the eye". Also it was written in *Ling Shu*: "The five *zang* and six *fu essences* flow into the eye and nourish it"; also "The twelve channels and 365 collaterals, *blood* and *qi* flow upward into the head and its orifices. Its *yang qi* essence flows into the eye to vitalize the eye."

Hua Tuo (?-208 A.D.), the famous Chinese medical physician and surgeon, had also proposed similar ideas for the eye in relationship to the whole body. In the 13th century, there was a book named *Yin Hai Jing Wei* (*Essentials of Ophthalmology*) with its authorship attributed to Sun Si-miao (581-682 A.D.). In the Ming Dynasty, physician Wang Kentang (1549-1613) wrote the book *Zheng Zhi Zhun Sheng* (*Guidelines in Syndrome Differentiation and Treatment*). He pointed out if the body has illness or disorder, the abnormal condition would reflect and show changes on the corresponding location of the eye. Another famous oculist Fu Ren-yu (also called Fu Yun-ke), who had more than 30 years clinical experience in treating eye diseases, wrote a book named *Shen Shi Yao Han*, also named as *Yan Ke Da Quan* (*A Complete Work of Ophthalmology*) during the Ming Dynasty 1644 A.D.[1]; its Volume 7 described eye diseases and listed 108 different eye conditions.

After many years of clinical practice, traditional Chinese medical doctors developed several therapeutic and theoretical systems about the eyes. These clinicians proved that the eye has a close relationship to the *zang-fu*. For example, the liver points to the eye and is the main organ affecting the eye and vision; gallbladder tends to have *damp heat* and transfers it to the liver. The heart dominates the *blood* and *mai*; the *blood* in the *mai* circulates throughout the whole body and flows to and nourishes the eye to enable clear vision; the small intestine is associated with *fire,* which influences the heart. When a person is healthy, the spleen *qi* flows upward to bring *qi* and *blood* to the eye. Since the stomach couples with spleen, they work together in the digestive process to produce nourishment and also manage the *blood*. The kidneys form the *source qi* and store *essence*, also associated with *water*. During aging, the kidney *qi* can weaken and may contribute to eye diseases. The bladder transforms fluid into urine and excretes it from the body. When disorders of the bladder appear, the fluid is retained in the tissues and manifests as swelling on the eyelids. The lungs govern *qi* and a person with sufficient *qi* shows a strong spirit and brightness in the eyes, with both pupils contracting and expanding smoothly and quickly. Collapsed lung *qi* presents as dull and damp on the eyes, with fixed dilation of the pupil. The large intestine excretes stool from the body, and if the transportation of the large intestine is weak, then *heat* will accumulate to cause *fire* that will rise up to influence the healthy eye.

Another system that affects the eyes is the meridians.[2] Of the twelve regular meridians, there are eight which have a direct relationship with the eye: Large Intestine, Stomach, Heart, Small Intestine, Urinary Bladder, Triple Warmer, Gallbladder, and Liver meridians. In four meridians - Lung, Spleen, Kidney and Pericardium - the *qi* does not flow directly to the eye but rather moves indirectly through internal and external relationships. The *qi* of the extra channels such as Du (Governing channel) runs between the two eyes while the Ren Mai (Conception channel) intersects the Stomach meridian at Chengji (St 1), allowing the *qi* to reach the eye. *Yang* Linking channel intersects with the Gallbladder meridian at Yangbai (GB 14), and the *Yin* Linking channel intersects at Tiantu (Co 22) and Lianquan (Co 23) on the Ren Mai, moving the *qi* up to the eye.

The Muscle (or Region) Channels, originating from the extremities and distributed under the skin, ascend to the head and trunk but do not actually reach the *zang-fu* organs. The muscle channels are similar to the twelve regular meridians in that they are divided into three hand *yin* and three hand *yang*, three foot *yin* and three foot *yang* channels. The relationship between these six *yang* muscle channels which all reach the head, along with the twelve regular meridians, form a complete network for allowing the *qi* and *blood* to flow up to the eyes for nourishment.

The ancient Chinese used another set of concepts for attempting to understand the world. Early traditional Chinese medical practitioners emphasized the importance of the Five Phases and Five Wheels (or Ring) Theories.[3] The Five Phases are *earth, fire, metal, wood and water;* the Five Wheels Theory is the application of the Five Phases for treatment of the eye. The Five Wheels Theory is that the *zang-fu* relates to certain parts of the eye anatomy and can therefore be used to define both the eye's anatomy and physiology.

(1) "Muscle Wheel"

(2) "Blood Wheel"

(3) "Energy Wheel"

(4) "Wind Wheel"

(5) "Water Wheel"

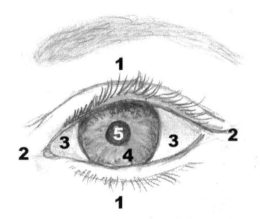

Figure 1 The Five Wheels: Relationships Between the Eye and the *Zang-Fu*

As shown in the above picture:

- *Rou* (flesh or muscle) Wheel is located on the upper and lower palpebrae, related to spleen and *earth* as the chief of Five Phases.
- *Xue* (*blood*) Wheel is located both at the inner and outer canthus of the eye, related to heart and *fire.*
- *Qi* (energy) Wheel is found on the white part of the eye (bulbar conjunctiva) and is related to lung and *metal.*
- *Feng* (*wind*) Wheel, located on the colored (dark brown, blue or green) part of the iris, is related to liver and *wood.*
- *Shui* (*water*) Wheel, located on the pupil, has colors of both black (when observed face to face) and clear (when a bright light is used for close examination) and relates to kidney and *water.*

In clinical practice, the Five Wheels of the eye are considered to be associated with five *zangs*. Therefore, the disorders of the five *zangs* reflect health conditions for corresponding locations of the eye for diagnosis, prevention and for treatment.

In 1970, the famous traditional Chinese physician, Professor Peng Jingshan of Liaoning TCM University, used the *bagua* (Eight Diagrams) and *baguo* (Eight Octants) Theories to develop a new ocular observation system and to adapt it for use in clinical treatment. This ocular diagnosis and periocular acupuncture technique rapidly spread throughout China and to other acupuncture centers of the world. Details of this system are described in Appendix One of this book.

You can see that the eye has a very close relationship to the body through the use of traditional Chinese medical theory, and that this type of medicine can offer effective benefits towards the prevention and treatment of eye diseases.

The focus of this book is on the most common conditions of aging eyes. There are ten chapters describing fifteen diseases or conditions. If not treated in the early stages, some of those diseases would end up needing surgical intervention. In traditional Chinese medicine, emphasis is placed upon prevention, called "*zhi wei bing*". Prevention methods for aging eye conditions, important for stopping early stage eye disease, include diet, self-massage, herbs and acupuncture. They can either prevent the development of, or slow down, the progression of eye disease so the senior can avoid undergoing surgery. This benefits not only the health of the senior, but also the families, society, and the economy.

Even though traditional Chinese medicine is very effective for the treatment of eye disease, there are two problems encountered by the practitioner. One of these is caused by the lack of using modern, high-tech methods to make a clear diagnosis of eye conditions or diseases. Because of the lack of advanced equipment, ancient practitioners did not actually understand the anatomy of the internal eye. They also could not offer a standard name for each eye disease since different practitioners gave a name for a condition based upon what he/she saw and thought. For example, Age-Related Macular Degeneration has many Chinese names including *Blurred Vision, Distorted Vision, Color Changed Vision, Cloud Moved to Eye, Sudden Blindness*, etc. This confusing situation created a large problem making it difficult to share the diagnosis of an eye disease with a patient, to discuss a finding with other practitioners, or to do advanced study and research. This is the reason we use the standard modern medical diagnostic names of eye diseases in this book.

A second weakness encountered when using traditional Chinese medicine for the treatment of eye disease, is that it is not effective in advanced stages and the patient typically needs to have surgery or other high tech treatments.

We hope that through the contents of this book, our readers will receive a clear knowledge and understanding of using traditional Chinese medicine for conditions of aging eyes, as well as the prevention and treatment of common eye diseases found in seniors.

References

[1] 漢英常用中醫藥詞彙, 謝竹藩, 黃孝楷主編, 北京醫學院, p. 424, 427, 443, 448, 462, 484, 490

[2] *Acupuncture---A Comprehensive Text*, Shanghai College of Traditional Medicine, Translated and Edited by John O'Connor and Dan Bensky, Eastland Press, Seattle, p. 47-73, 90-99

[3] *Window of Health---Ocular Diagnosis and Periocular Acupuncture*, Compiled by Hoy Ping Yee Chan, Northwest Institute of Acupuncture & Oriental Medicine, 1996, Seattle, p. 2-3, 13-37

CHAPTER TWO

Eye Examination

The key focus of the basic eye examination on a senior patient is observation; thus the eye exam begins the moment the patient walks into the office. The Chinese medical practitioner should pay attention to the following conditions when they first meet a patient.

Basic Eye Examination for Senior Patients

- Watch the patient as he/she walks into your room. How is the posture of his or her walk? Does the patient need someone at his/her side to help or guide the way?

- Look at patient's *shen*, emphasized in the eyes: Is the *shen* of the eyes sharp or dull? Is the reflex of the eyes fast or slow? Is there emotion in the eyes? Is the face natural or depressed?

- It is important to check the patient's vision before you examine his/her eyes. Vision (visual acuity) is measured by using the familiar Snellen Chart, which has lines of increasingly smaller letters. Each line of the chart corresponds to a different level of vision.

- Check the patient's blood pressure.

Eye Observation Based on Western Medicine[1]

Distance Vision Testing: The patient stands at a distance of 20 feet away from the wall where the Snellen Eye Chart hangs. If an exam room is not big enough for this distance, you can use a mirror to reflect the necessary length for a total of 20 feet. Record the vision using a fraction.

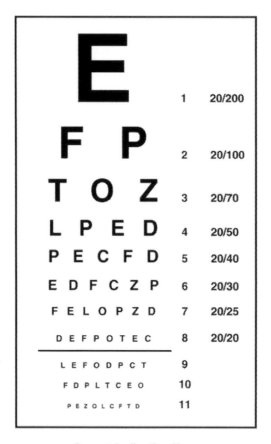

Figure 2 Snellen Eye Chart

The top number of the fraction represents the testing distance from the chart, so it is always written as 20. The bottom number represents the smallest line the patient can see, meaning the patient must correctly read more than three letters on that line. Check each eye separately. Test the right eye first by covering the left eye and recording the vision; then cover the right eye and check the left. You also have to understand the abbreviations used by ophthalmologists: the "OD" represents right eye; the "OS" represents left eye; and the "OU" represents both eyes.

If the right eye can see only the large letter at the top of the chart, the record is designated as 20/200. If the left eye can see the smallest letters on the line directly above the bottom line on the chart, the record is designated as 20/20. This is considered to be normal vision. This result indicates that the patient using his left eye only and standing a distance of 200 feet can see the letter on the top line, while his right eye can see the same letter at 20 feet.

If the patient cannot even see the letter on the top line, then use your fingers to check. Stand at some estimated distance first and ask the patient to count how many fingers you are holding up. If the patient cannot see them, move closer until he/she can actually count the fingers (CF). The findings are recorded as: Fingers/ ? feet or ? inches.

If the patient cannot see the fingers approximately 2 inches in front of his/her eye, then ask if he/she can see the moving hand, noting how far the distance is from the eye. Record your findings as: Hand Motion (HM) /? inches or ? cm.

If the patient cannot see the moving hand, go to a dark room, and, using a candle or hand light, ask the patient to point out where the light is coming from. Check the farthest distance and record as Light Perception (LP)/ ? feet or ? inches.

You also need to check if the pupil has any light reaction and record as LR (+) or (-).

Close Vision Testing: Some patients need his/her close vision checked. Hold the chart 16 inches away from the eye and ask the patient to read the smallest letters on the chart that he/she can see and then record; check right eye first, then the left eye.

Relative Terms of Normal Eye Anatomy and Physiological Functions[1, 2]

Before moving on to the actual eye exam, we will briefly review the anatomy of the normal eye.

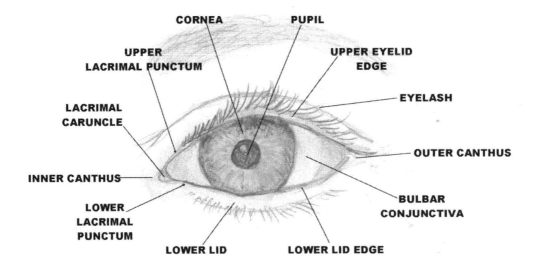

Figure 3 Normal Anatomy, Left Eye, Frontal View

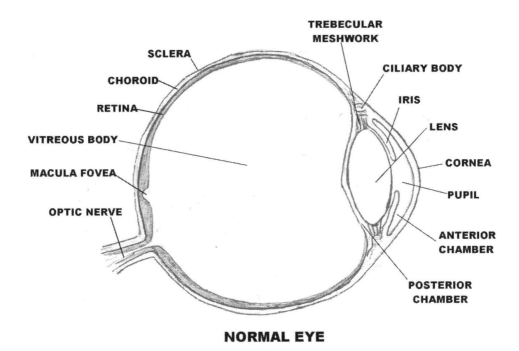

Figure 4 Normal Eye Anatomy, Side View

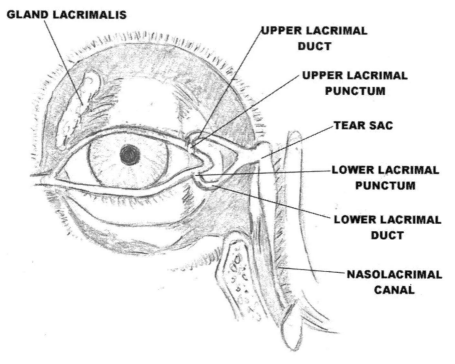

Figure 5 Lacrimal Apparatus, Right Eye

- Cornea: The outer part of the anterior eye. It is a transparent membrane which does not contain any blood vessels but has plenty of sensitive nerves from the eye branch of the fifth cranial nerve. The diameter of the cornea is normally 9-12.5 mm.
- Pupil: When seen through the center of the cornea, it is an adjustable round opening which allows light to enter the eye. The normal size is from 2.5 – 4 mm but it can be from 0.5 to 9 mm.
- Iris: The iris is the colored ring of tissue behind the cornea. In the center of the iris is the pupil. The iris contains a circle-like sphincter muscle which is controlled by the parasympathetic nerves. When it contracts, the pupil shrinks smaller. In contrast, it has another muscle which is controlled by the sympathetic nerve to dilate the pupil. When the pupil is stimulated by light, the pupil shrinks, a reaction called the pupil light reflex or LR (light reaction). In the dark, the pupil automatically enlarges.

The function of the iris is to regulate the amount of light entering the eye by adjusting the size of the pupil.

- **Ciliary Body:** This extends from the root of the iris and produces the aqueous humor from its anterior part called the ciliary process. The posterior portion, called pars plana or orbiculus ciliaris, is like a flat ring. The ciliary body also manages the refractive power of the lens.
- **Lens:** A crystalline and resilient structure, the lens is seen behind the pupil. The lens, suspended on the back of the iris and in front of the vitreous, helps to focus the light rays on the retina. The lens does not have blood vessels, but is nourished by the aqueous humor. With aging, the nucleus of the lens becomes bigger and harder and its resilience reduces causing presbyopia, an inability to focus on nearby objects.
- **Anterior Chamber:** This is the space found between the cornea, iris and lens that contains the aqueous humor.
- **Posterior Chamber:** This space is behind the iris, surrounded by the ciliary body and the equatorial part of the lens. The aqueous humor starts to flow from here.
- **Aqueous Humor:** Produced by the ciliary processes, this watery transparent fluid circulates from the posterior chamber through the pupil, flows into the anterior chamber past the trabecular meshwork and Schlemm Canal, and finally goes into the aqueous humor vein network and forward towards the ciliary anterior vein.
- **Schlemm Canal:** The canal is located at the corner of the anterior chamber where the aqueous humor drains from the anterior chamber into the vein network of the sclera.
- **Trabecular Meshwork:** A supportive fiber of sponge-like connective tissue resembling a small beam extending from the side of cornea and located at the medial side of the Schlemm Canal. Its function is to block any micro-material bodies in the aqueous humor so they cannot leave the anterior chamber and move into the Schlemm Canal, thus keeping the aqueous humor flowing freely.
- **Vitreous Chamber:** Found behind the eye lens, this cavity is filled with vitreous humor to hold the eye's shape against outside pressure.

- **Vitreous Humor (body):** The transparent gelatinous substance that fills the vitreous chamber. Since there are no blood vessels in the vitreous humor, nutrition comes from the aqueous humor and choroid. Because of this, if a person's metabolism is very low, there is not enough nourishment and the vitreous humor becomes more liquid or turns to string-like scars. The vitreous humor cannot be replenished and if damaged, can lead to retinal detachment.
- **Retina:** The light-sensitive layer of tissue located in the back of the eye that receives images which are transmitted to the brain via the optic nerve. One layer of the retina contains rods and cones.
- **Macula:** A minute yellowish area located at the center of the retina of the eye, where visual perception is most acute. At the center of the macula is a tiny 1-3 mm depression called the fovea centralis (foveola)[3] that provides shape, clear and straight-ahead vision.
- **Choroid:** The vascular layer of the eye containing connective tissue; the choroid is found between the retina and the sclera.
- **Optic Nerve:** The bundle of nerve fibers at the back of the eye that carries visual messages from the retina to the brain.
- **Sclera:** The tough outer layer of the eye that protects the entire eyeball.

Examination of the Palpebrae[4]

The palpebrae, or eyelids, are protective layers of skin, muscles and tissue that surround the anterior surface of the eyes. Their basic function is to prevent the eyes from being injured by the entry of foreign materials like dust and debris, or from bright lights that could permanently ruin the eyes. The eyelids are also useful in keeping the eyes well lubricated by producing and spreading tears and mucus evenly across the eyeballs.

The palpebrae for each eye are composed of two lids: an upper eyelid that extends upwards from the eye towards the eyebrow, and a lower eyelid that descends from the eye towards the cheek. The anatomy of the eyelid includes important structures such as the skin, hypodermis, levator palpebrae muscle, orbicularis oculi muscle, orbital septum, tarsal plates, glands, blood vessels, nerves and conjunctiva.

Examination of the palpebrae includes the following:

- Shape: Is there any swelling, scars, damage, are both sides even?
    - Movement: Both eyelids should normally open and close at the same time with a smooth and even movement, as well as close tightly.
    - Border:
        - Upper Part: The superior border of the upper eyelid is distinct where it meets the eyebrow at the orbit.
        - Lower Part: The inferior border of the lower eyelid is not nearly as distinct as the superior in relation to the orbit due to layers of soft tissue.
- Palpebral Margin: The free edge of the palpebra, where the eyelashes emerge.
- The Skin of the Eyelid: This is the thinnest skin on the body. It is very flexible and easily stretched and therefore very easily wrinkled. Both connective and fatty tissues are located immediately under the skin. Muscle tissue is located beneath the connective tissue layer.
- Palpebral Conjunctiva: The interior part of the eyelid.

Examination of the Exterior Portion of the Anterior Eye[5]

There is no need to routinely check the color of the mucous membrane lining the inside of the eyelid unless there are obvious problems since it is very uncomfortable to evert the eyelid to make this observation.

Note that the colors listed below refer to the entire conjunctiva and not just the capillaries.

Bulbar Conjunctiva Colors

- White: Natural white is a healthy color, considered normal.

- **Yellow:** The color is on the sclera, but actually looks like it is on the conjunctiva. Bright yellow relates to *damp heat* in the liver or gallbladder. Faded yellow relates to *cold damp*.
- **Pink:** Relates to lung, allergy, overwork, fatigue, lack of sleep (*yin* deficiency) as well as other eye diseases.
- **Red:** Relates to lung or heart, infection, extreme fatigue, fever (excess *heat* or even excess *fire*); other eye diseases.
- **Grey/Blue:** Indicates weakness or some chronic health condition and may relate to kidney internal *cold* or *wind*. Note that some healthy children can have a light blue color but, at the same time, the conjunctiva looks bright and shiny.

If there is a blood clot or subconjunctival hemorrhage under the membrane making it impossible to ascertain the color of the bulbar conjunctiva, the practitioner needs to identify where the blood is coming from by asking the patient more related questions, such as, "Any coughing? Heavy lifting? Any injury especially to the face or eye?" According to Chinese medicine, clots are related to *blood* stagnancy from the spleen.

Another standard eye exam performed by Western medical doctors is to locate the exact area of redness. This can be important since the treatment protocols for problems in the two areas are very different; knowing where the problem stems from allows the practitioner to give the most appropriate treatment for a patient's specific condition.

Location of the redness

- **Ciliary congestion** - Redness appearing around the border of the cornea. If found within 4mm of the anterior conjunctiva, it is indicative of more severe eye disease such as keratitis, irisitis, etc. If this condition is observed it requires immediate attention and the patient should be sent to an ophthalmologist since the iris needs treatment and the pupil may need to be dilated - a procedure not routinely performed by traditional Chinese medical practitioners. The blood supply for this area is the anterior ciliary artery.

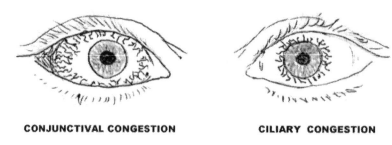

Figure 6 Conjunctival (L) vs. Ciliary Congestion (R)

- Conjunctival Congestion - Redness appearing on the exterior conjunctiva around the edge of the eyeball indicates that just the external eye has a condition such as conjunctivitis. The blood supply for this area is the palpebral internal artery. Acupuncturists can get fast and excellent results working on this condition.

Ocular Observation of the Pathological Changes of the Capillary Branches of the Bulbar Conjunctiva (From Professor Peng's *Observation of Changing Conditions of the Whole Body*)

- Broad stalks: Observed in stubborn cases.

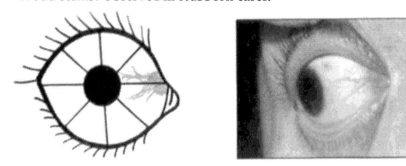

Figure 7 Broad Stalk, Enlarged and Prolonged

- Abnormally swollen, enlarged, prolonged and twisted: The stage of disease is severe and the illness is an excess condition.

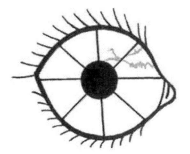 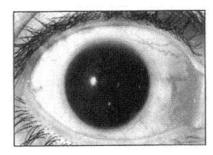

Figure 8 Abnormally Twisted

- **Branches beyond ocuzone boundaries:** Illness is in more than one organ.

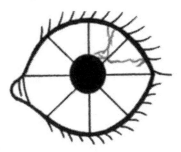 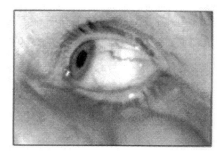

Figure 9 Branches Beyond the Ocuzone Boundaries

- **Divided into branches:** Usually located under the pupil, indicating a variable illness that easily changes to different symptoms.

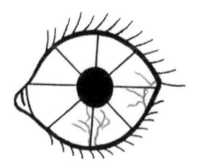 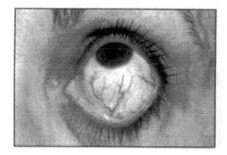

Figure 10 Divided into Branches

- **Capillaries standing out or as a raised line of protrusion:** Illness is located in the six *fu* organs.

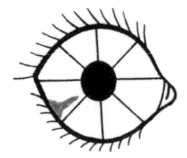 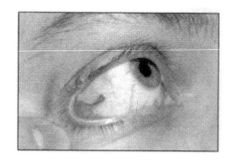

Figure 11 Capillaries Standing Out

- **Diamond-like shape:** Indicates an illness with complicated symptoms.

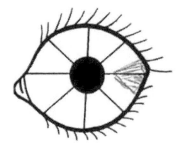 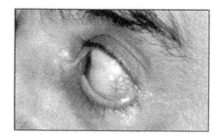

Figure 12 Diamond-Like Shape

- **Indistinct region:** This is usually observed in the liver-gallbladder zone, with symptoms of tension, stress and depression.

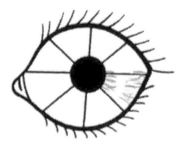 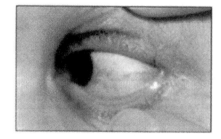

Figure 13 Indistinct Region

- **Projection as a dew drop:** If it shows on the stomach and/or intestine regions, the projection points to parasitic infection. If it appears in other regions, it may be blood stagnation.

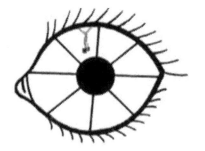 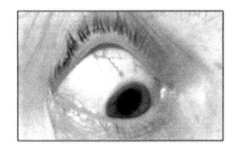

Figure 14 Projecting as a Dew Drop

Color Variances in the Capillary Branches

Note that these colors apply only to the color of the capillaries, not the entire conjunctiva (as discussed on page 14, *Colors of the Bulbar Conjunctiva*).

- Shades of Red
    - True red: Onset of illness and excessive condition.
    - Purple-red: More feverish illness.
    - Dark red: Illness invades into organs, fever is progressing.
    - Black in with red: *Heat* developing disorder.
    - Yellow in with red: Illness getting better.
- Shades of Gray
    - Faded gray: Weakness of *qi*, lack of *blood* or *cold* condition of *qi* or *blood* stagnation.
    - True gray: An old illness.
- Shades of Yellow
    - Yellowish: Rate of improvement yet to be determined.

References

[1] *The Crystal Clear Guide to Sight for Life*, by Johnny L. Gayton, M.D. et al., Starburst Publisher, Lancaster, PA, U.S.A. 1996, p. 52-53

[2] 眼科學, 毛文書主編, 人民衛生出版社, 北京, p. 17-25

[3] American Health Assistance Foundation. Retrieved from http://www.ahaf.org

[4] 現代眼科手冊, 楊鈞主編, 人民衛生出版社, p. 41-45

[5] *Window of Health---Ocular Diagnosis and Periocular Acupuncture*, Compiled by Hoy Ping Yee Chan, Northwest Institute of Acupuncture & Oriental Medicine, Seattle, 1996, p. 5-12; 45-48

CHAPTER THREE

Blepharoptosis and Myasthenia

Blepharoptosis

Shang Bao Xia Chui (Upper Eyelid Dropped Down)
Qin Feng (*Wind* Invaded)
Jian Fei (Useless Eyelid)

Blepharoptosis, or ptosis for short, is a condition in which usually both upper eyelids sag, possibly interfering with vision. The disorder is most commonly seen in elderly people as the muscle fibers in both eyelids naturally weaken with advancing age. The condition can deteriorate if there is lack of sleep or fatigue in the afternoon. Newborns can be affected by ptosis in both eyes due to kidney *essence* deficiency causing genetic defect. Children and young adults can also experience blepharoptosis but in one eye only due to severe infection, eye injury, or tumor. In this book, we will focus on blepharoptosis in the senior.

Causes of Blepharoptosis in Seniors[1]

Spleen *qi* deficiency prevents the *yang qi* from rising, resulting in a lack of power to lift up the eyelid. If the spleen *qi* fails to move and transform the *qi*, *damp* obstruction and *phlegm* development can occur. Then *wind-phlegm* blocks the network vessels (*luo mai*) with a resultant slowing down and weakening of movement of the eyelid's muscles, finally causing the eyelids to drop down.

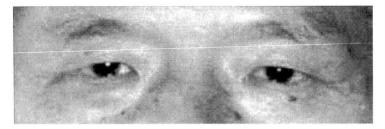

Figure 15 Example of Early Stage Blepharoptosis: Both Eyelids Sag

Examination

When both eyes are looking straight forward, the margin of the upper eyelid normally covers the top 1/5 of the upper portion of the cornea (not beyond 3 mm), which means the margin of this eyelid cannot go beyond the 10 to 2 o'clock position.

Blepharoptosis is indicated if the upper eyelid extends beyond 3mm from the upper edge of the cornea. In a severe case, it may fully cover the cornea. Looking at this type of patient's face, the hairs of the eyebrows will appear straight and there will be many winkles on the forehead from his/her efforts to keep the eyelids up. When the space between the upper and lower eye margins is narrower than normal (average is 7.54 mm), it indicates the upper eyelid has dropped.

Symptoms

Based on the above mentioned exam, in some cases, patients often need to raise their head, lift up their eyebrows, or even use their fingers to lift up an eyelid to help them see better.

However, there are some seniors who look like their eyelids are drooping because they have very loose skin on their eyebrows and eyelids. A simple way to rule out the disease of ptosis is to have them use two fingers to lift up the upper eyelid and check if the margin is still at the normal limit (less than 3mm). Another method is to use a finger and apply pressure at the middle of the eyebrow to check if, when the eyeball moves upward, the upper eyelid is able to lift up. This finding means that the patient does not have a ptosis diagnosis.

If the ptosis occurs suddenly in only one eye, it is most likely caused by the paralysis of the oculomotor nerve (3rd cranial nerve). Further medical examination is needed to exclude the conditions of tumor, stroke, diabetes or injury.

TCM Differential Diagnosis and Treatment[2]

Herbal Treatment
The first formula is based on the Five Wheels Theory.

Spleen *Qi* Deficiency

Treatment Principle	Tonify the spleen *yang* and boost *qi*
Formula 1	Bu Zhong Yi Qi Tang---Codonopsis (Ginseng) & Astragalus Combination[3]
	Huang Qi, Dang Shen, Zhi Gan Cao, Dang Gui, Chen Pi, Sheng Ma, Chai Hu, Bai Zhu

Formulas #2 and #3 are based on Eight Principles Syndromes and Six Excessive of Atmospheric Influences.

Deficiency of *Qi* and *Blood*; *Wind Evil* Entering the Vessels (*Luo Mai*)

Treatment Principle	Dispel *wind* and boost *qi* to nourish *blood* flow
Formula 2	Ren Shen Yang Rong (Ying) Tang---Ginseng & Rehmannia Combination[4]
	Dang Gui, Bai Shao, Shou Di Huang, Dang Shen, Bai Zhu, Fu Ling, Zhi Gan Cao, Rou Gui, Wu Wei Zi, Yuan Zhi, Chen Pi, Da Zao, Huang Qi
For severe cases to expel *wind* faster add	Qin Jiao, Tao Ren, *Di Long, *Jiang Can

Herbs with an asterisk (*) indicate an animal product

Wind-Phlegm Obstructs the Vessels

Treatment Principle	To control *wind* and expel *phlegm*; quicken the *blood* flow and clear the vessels
Formula 3	Zheng Rong Tang---Reforming Face Formula[5]
	Qiang Huo, #Bai Fu Zi, Fang Feng, Qin Jiao, #Dan (Ting) Nan Xing, #Ban Xia, *Jiang Can, Mu Gua, Gan Cao, Sheng Jiang, Huang Song Jie
For a chronic case, to quicken blood flow and dispel stasis add	Dan Shen, Chuan Xiong, Si Gua Luo, San Qi, *Di Long

Herbs marked with a pound sign (#) are slightly poisonous. These types of herbs are only used in small doses so the formulas are safe.

Acupuncture Treatment

In general, for the treatment of any eye disease with acupuncture, do treatments twice weekly with 10 treatments constituting one course. Choose *either* ocuzone points or filiform needling for the treatment. Note that seven star needling is good to do at any time or in combination with either the ocuzone or filiform techniques.

Acupuncture treatment selections for specific eye conditions will be given in each chapter.

For treating a light case of ptosis or one in its early stage, only use acupuncture treatment as herbs are not needed. Running needle is the most effective acupuncture approach.

For any acupuncture technique always include: Baihui (GV 20).

Running Needles:

Zanzhu (BL 2) ----------> Yuyao (M-HN-6 extra point)

Yangbai (GB 14) -------> Yuyao

Sizhukong (TB 23) -----> Yuyao

Taiyang (M-HN-9 extra Point) ----> Tongziliao (GB 1)

Zusanli (ST 36) and Sanyinjiao (SP 6) should be added to any of the above combinations. (Note that these are not running needles).

Filiform Needles: Choose from one of two alternate groups of points:

Group 1: Zanzhu (BL 2), Yangbai (GB 14), Taiyang (M-HN-9), Zusanli (ST 36), Sanyinjiao (SP 6).

Group 2: Yuyao (M-HN-6), Shangxing (GV 23), Muchuang (GB 16), Sizhukong (TB 23), Qihai (CO 6), Hegu (LI 4).

Ocular Needles: Ocuzones Upper Warmer (Zone 5), Spleen (Zone 11).

Note that during ocular observation if you can see some changes in the capillaries in particular ocuzones, add those to zones 5 and 11 or choose the zones with observed changes instead.

Seven Star Needles: Seven Star needling is done following other ptosis treatments. For best results, it is helpful if the patient has a family member who can be taught to do seven star needle tapping for them between visits.

Tap on Five Back Shu Points: Feishu (BL 13), Xinshu (BL 15), Ganshu (BL 18), Pishu (BL 20), Shenshu (BL 23).

The patient can also gently tap on the acupuncture points around his/her eye orbit. Note that this area is very sensitive so the tapping should be gradually increased as tolerated and only up to the point where it still feels comfortable.

Ear Needles: Use press tack needles or magnetic pellets on the ear if the patient cannot come in for treatments as often as desired. Use filiform needles for 30 minutes, then remove and replace them with pellets held with ear tape. The patient should leave the pellets on until he/she feels irritation and can then remove them.

Select Ear Points: Eye, Lung, Spleen, Heart, Kidney

Moxibustion: Used by the patient to supplement his/her other treatments. In the early stage of the disease, moxibustion can be used as a preventive treatment. Remember to use moxa with caution in post-menopausal women or persons with severe *yin* deficiency.

Xuehai (SP 10), Zusanli (ST 36); or

Feishu (BL 13), Pishu (BL 20); or

Baihui (GV 20), Qihai (CO 6)

Prevention and Diet

It is most important for the patient to do self-care massage and moxibustion. Teach them and it can help to delay the progression of eye disease for as long as they live.

The principle for prevention is to supplement the spleen *yang* and *blood*, and keep boosting strong lung *qi* to prevent *wind* invasion.

Self-Care Massage: Knocking on the head; massaging around the orbital edges and ears. Details can be found in Chapter 13, General Prevention for Aging Eyes.

Also massage the Back Shu points; soles of the feet and Yongquan (KI 1).

Moxibustion: Use indirect moxa on Zusanli (ST 36) and Xuehai (SP 10).

Diet

Treatment Principle	Tonify spleen *qi*
	Shan Yao Bu Pi Congee
	Shan Yao 15 gram + rice 100 gram
Treatment Principle	Tonify *Blood*
All foods can be added to Shan Yao with rice to make congee	Ou Jie Bu XueTang
	Lotus node (Ou Jie) 1 lb without core, Red Date (Hong Zao) 10 pieces. Dry Longan fruit (Long Yan Rou) 15 -30 gm.

Myasthenia Gravis

(May count as one type of *Wei Zheng*)

Modern medical science considers the cause of myasthenia to be due to the degeneration of acetylcholine receptors (AchR) resulting from the obstruction of the transmission between the nerves and muscles. At the onset of myasthenia, the first symptom that appears is drooping on both upper eyelids. Myasthenia, which also affects other muscles in the body, differs from blepharoptosis where there is no muscle weakness involved other than in the eyelids.

Signs and Symptoms

Myasthenia is a disease which affects the voluntary muscles of the entire body. In Western medicine it is labeled an autoimmune system disease. However, the true pathogenesis is still not clear. It may be caused by a malfunction in the transference of signals from the nerve to the muscle. Onset usually is very slow and starts in the upper eyelids. Symptoms include weakness of the voluntary muscles and having muscles fatigue easily if doing repetitive moves such as continuously blinking the eyelids. This would be hard for a myasthenia patient to do although after taking a rest, the patient would be able to resume blinking his/her eyelids again without difficulty.

Eventually weakness will move down to other muscles and the patient can have a difficult time chewing or swallowing. Weakness can also appear in the limbs. The disease can also create a worse condition, that of breathing difficulty, which would need emergency care.

It is important for an acupuncturist to differentiate this disease from blepharoptosis, which only affects the eyelids. For myasthenia treatment, an acupuncturist should work with the patient's physician, who may use Western medicine such as Prostigmin for intramuscular injection. 15-30 minutes following the injection, the upper eyelids are able to lift up like normal for a while.[6]

TCM Differential Diagnosis and Treatment

Diagnostic Key: Usually the onset of this disease is at a young age, but in some cases the symptoms are concealed. Use the finger technique to check the upper eyelid to see if it can be raised. Also check the myodynamic strength (muscular contraction) of the patient's forearm.

Herbal Treatment

Spleen *Qi* Deficiency

Treatment Principle	Tonify spleen *yang*
Formula 1	Bu Zhong Yi Qi Tang

Spleen & Kidney *Yang* Deficiency

Treatment Principle	Tonify the spleen and kidney *yang*
Formula 4	Fu Gui Li Zhong Tang---Aconite, Ginseng & Ginger Combination[7]
	#Fu Zi, Rou Gui, Gan Jiang, Ren Shen, Bai Zhu, Zhi Gan Cao

Acupuncture Treatment

- Use blepharoptosis points; you may add more points on the *yangming* channels and five Back Shu points.
- Use moxa on the five back shu points.
- Special technique He Gu Cui[8] (see below) - using Yuyao as the first insertion point.

The He Gu Ci Technique Using One Needle

1. Insert perpendicularly into the superficial muscle layer at extra point Yuyao (M-HN-6), located in the center of the eyebrow.
2. Pull the needle out to just beneath the skin and insert horizontally towards Zanzhu (BL 2) and obtain *qi*.

3. Pull the needle out to just beneath the skin and turn the needle laterally towards Sizhukong (TW23) and obtain *qi*.

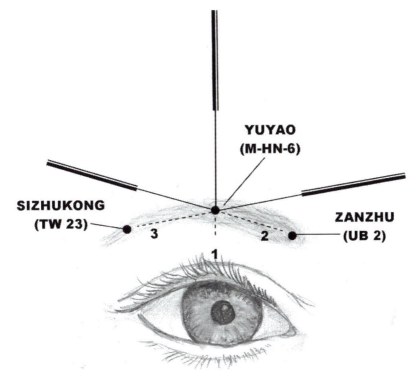

Figure 16 He Gu Zi Technique Using One Needle

Note that this technique is usually only used in the thicker muscle area; for eye treatment it is inserted more at about 15 - 20 degree horizontal angle (as shown in the drawing) due to local anatomy.

References

[1] 中醫眼科學, 廖品正主編, 人民衛生出版社, p. 146-148

[2] 中醫眼科學, 廣卅中醫學院主編, 上海科學技術出版社, p. 45-46

[3] Formula 1: 補中益氣湯, 中醫眼科學, 廖品正主編, 人民衛生出版社, p. 343, #94

[4] Formula 2: 人參養榮湯, Ibid., p. 338, #16

[5] Formula 3: 正容湯, Ibid., p. 340, #36

[6] 現代眼科手冊, 楊鈞主編, 人民衛生出版社, p. 297

[7] Formula 4: 附桂理中湯, 中醫眼科學, 廣卅中醫學院主編, 上海科學技術出版社, p. 126, #129 + 附子, 肉桂

[8] 合谷刺法為主治療眼肌型重症肌無47例, 馮起國等, 中國針灸, 1998年, 第1期, p. 33-34

CHAPTER FOUR

Dry Eye

Shen Shui Jiang Ke (Tears Almost Dried Out)

A normal eye is always moist because it constantly bathes itself in a slow, steady rate of tears. If this does not happen, or if environmental conditions cause increased tear film evaporation, the condition is called dry eye. This can result in chronic irritation leading to inflammation of the tarsus of the eye and blepharitis marginalis. Dry eye is also described by the medical term keratitis sicca, which generally means a decreased quality or quantity of tears. Ophthalmologists may use the Schirmer test to see if the amount of tearing is at normal range. Also they may check how long it takes the tear film to break. The shorter the time for a tear to evaporate, the more severe the symptom. Dry eye is not considered to be a disease on its own but is a syndrome that includes a whole group of symptoms.

Causes of Dry Eye[1,2]

Dry eye basically results when there is decreased secretion - both in quantity and quality - from the lacrimal glands. The most common cause of dry eyes is the normal aging process, especially associated with post-menopausal women. It may also occur as a result of other health conditions or as a side effect of many medications such as antihistamines, antidepressants, certain blood pressure medicines, Parkinson's medications or birth control pills. Home or office air conditioning or a dry heat system can also cause the eyes to dry out. Another cause is insufficient blinking, such as when a person stares at a computer screen or iPad all day. Recently, dry eye symptoms are developing in more people at a younger age (under 40 years old and often even extending to children) due to prolonged viewing on the computer, watching television, playing games on an iPad or wearing contact lenses.

Symptoms[1,2]

The most common symptoms of dry eye include uncomfortable dryness in the eyes, stinging, itching, scratchiness, a feeling of something foreign in the eye, a burning sensation, redness or sticky mucous around the eyelashes in the morning. Some patients also complain about having eye fatigue, vision that varies - sometimes better, sometimes not, dry mouth, tearing, fear of facing into the wind, afraid to look at fluorescent lights, and even joint pain.

Dry eye rarely causes blindness, but it can affect the quality or sharpness of vision. When a dry eye patient constantly lives with fatigued and irritated eyes, this can raise stress levels and limit activities like reading and driving. Damage to the cornea caused by rubbing eyes too often can also cause keratitis or corneal ulcer, leading to a nebula or scar on the cornea with resultant loss of visual acuity.

TCM Differential Diagnosis and Treatment[3]

Traditional Chinese medicine states that a deficiency of *qi* and *yin* will decrease the amount of nutrition nourishing the eyes, resulting in dryness and a scratchy feeling in them. There are five deficiency patterns.

Liver *Qi* Depression and Liver *Yin* Deficiency

Symptoms: Dryness in the eyes may appear with mental and emotional depression, sleeplessness, fatigue, loss of appetite, loss of interest for doing normal activities, fear of noise and light or meeting people, and body weakness.

Herbal Treatment[4]

Treatment Principle	Soothe the liver and nourish *blood*; boost *qi* and nourish *yin*
Formula 5 Formula 6	Xiao Yao San---Dang Gui & Bupleurum Combination Powder[5] + Sheng Mai San---Engender Pulse Powder[6]
	Chai Hu, Bai Zhu, Bai Shao, Dang Gui, Fu Ling, Zhi Gan Cao, Bo He, Wei Jiang + Ren Shen, Mai Dong, Wu Wei Zi

Acupuncture Treatment

Ocular Needles: Ocuzones Upper Warmer (Zone 5) and Liver (Zone 6); or use Heart (Zone 9); or you can choose other points based on observed changes in other ocuzones.

Along with the use of the ocular needles, add in:

Filiform Needles: Qimen (LR 14), Neiguan (PC 6); or Shanzhong (Ren 17), Taichong (LR 3).

Lung *Yin* Deficiency and Lung Hidden *Heat* (Deep-Lying *Fire*)

Symptoms: Uncomfortable dryness in the eyes, patient blinks often, no redness or swelling, the eyes are dull. The patient also presents with dryness in the nose, throat and mouth, red tongue with dry coat, fine and rapid pulse.

Herbal Treatment

Treatment Principle	Clear lung *heat* and nourish lung *yin*
Formula 7	Sang Bai Pi Tang---Mulberry Bark Formula[7]
	Sang Bai Pi, Ze Xie, Xuan Shan, Gan Cao, Mai Dong, Huang Qin, Ju Hua, Di Gu Pi, Jie Geng, Fu Ling
Also add supporting herbs	Sheng Di Huang, Tian Hua Fen, Shi Hu

Acupuncture Treatment

Ocular Needles: Ocuzones Lung (Zone 1), Upper Warmer (Zone 5); or Heart (Zone 9); or you can choose other points based on observed changes in other ocuzones.

Along with the use of the ocular needles, add in:

Filiform Needles: Chize (LU 5), Neiguan (PC 6).

Liver-Kidney *Yin* Deficiency

Symptoms: Uncomfortable dryness, fatigued eyes often leading to closing the eyelids, dryness of the mouth and throat, red tongue without coating, fine pulse.

Herbal Treatment

Treatment Principle	Enrich and nourish liver and kidney *yin*
Formula 8	Qi Ju Di Huang Wan---Lycium, Chrysanthemum & Rehmannia Formula[8]
	Gou Qi Zi, Ju Hua, Shou Di Huang, Shan Zhu Yu, Shan Yao, Ze Xie, Mu Dan Pi, Fu Ling

Acupuncture Treatment

Ocular Needles: Ocuzones Kidney (Zone 3), Upper Warmer (Zone 5), Liver (Zone 6).

Along with the use of the ocular needles, add in:

Filiform Needles: Sanyinjiao (SP 6) or Xingjian (LR 2), Taixi (KI 3).

Fluid and Tear Shortage

Symptoms: Dryness with pain when the eyelids open and close, the surface of the eye ball is without moisture, and there is a typical shiny, red tongue.

Herbal Formula

Treatment Principle	Nourish *yin* and engender liquid
Formula 9	Zeng Ye Tang---Increase Liquid Formula[9]
	Xuan Shen, Mai Dong, Sheng Di Huang
For enhancing *yin* add	Sha Shen and Yu Zhu

Acupuncture Treatment

Ocular Needles: Ocuzones Lung (Zone 1), Kidney (Zone 3), Upper Warmer (Zone 5).

Along with the use of the ocular needles, add in:

Filiform Needles: Sanyinjiao (SP 6) or Taiyuan (LU 9), Taixi (KI 3).

Lung-Spleen *Damp-Heat*

Symptoms: Heavy feeling of the eyelids, dryness and a feeling like sand in the eyes, no redness on the white of the eye but may have redness and thickness on the conjunctival portion of the eyelid.

Herbal Treatment

Treatment Principle	Clear lung and spleen *damp heat*, tonify the spleen and inhibit the dampness
Formula 10 NOTE: This formula cannot be taken too long	Chu Shi Tang---Clear Dampness Formula[10]
	Lian Qiao, Hua Shi, Che Qian Zi, Zhi Ke, Huang Qin, Huang Lian, Mu Tong, Chen Pi, Jing Jie, Fu Ling, Fang Feng, Gan Cao
Add herbs for producing fluid	Xuan Shan, Shi Hu, Lu Gen, Sheng Di Huang, Mai Men Dong

Acupuncture Treatment

Ocular Needles: Ocuzones Lung (Zone 1), Upper Warmer (Zone 5), Spleen (Zone 11)

Along with the use of the ocular needles, add in:

Filiform Needles: Sanyinjiao (SP 6), Fenglong (ST 40).

Special Formula Ba Zhen Tang[11]

In clinical practice, some traditional Chinese and Western eye doctors prefer to use Western medical examination to diagnose dry eye. Also, rather than using traditional Chinese medical identification to select a treatment approach, they use only one herbal formula for treatment. The base formula is Ba Zhen Tang but additional herbs may be added or removed depending on each patient's specific condition.

Treatment Principle	Tonify *qi* and *blood*, harmonize *yin* and *yang*
Formula 11 (This formula combines two common formulas: Si Wei Tang - also named Si Jun Zi Tang - and Si Wu Tang.)	Ba Zhen Tang---Angelica and Ginseng Eight Combination[12]
	Si Wei Tang[13]: Dang Shen, Fu Ling, Bai Zhu, Zhi Gan Cao; Si Wu Tang[13]: Dang Gui, Bai Shao, Shou Di Huang, Chuan Xiong
For enhancing *qi* and expelling *wind heat* you may also add	Huang Qi; Ju Hua, Jing Jie, Fang Feng, Gu Jing Cao (remove Bai Zhu and Zhi Gan Cao)

Formulas Used for External Treatment of Dry Eye[14]

Formula A

- Use for *yin* deficiency causing dry eyes.
- Herbs: Shi Hu, Sha Shen, Ju Hua, Gou Qi, Mi Meng Hua.
- Cook until it starts to steam.

Formula B

- Use for *wind heat* causing eye pain.
- Herbs: Shi Chang Pu, Man Jing Zi.
- Put in pot and cook until steam starts rising, then add Bo He.

Formula C

- Use for dry eye with excess *heat* or *fire* pattern.
- Herbs: Fang Feng, Jing Jie, Pu Gong Ye.
- Put in a pot and cook until almost to a boil, then add Bo He and continuing cooking until it starts to steam.

Method for Using the Above Formulas

Note that if the patient is hospitalized, he/she can use a nebulizer. For home care the patient can use a thermos mug by following these directions:

1. After cooking the herbs, place them in a thermos mug that has a 1.5 inch diameter opening.
2. Using thick paper or a plastic shield, cut a hole of the same 1.5 inch diameter, so that as the steam comes up through the hole it will not spread to the sides of the face but instead is focused on the eyelids.
3. The patient needs to close both eyelids and self adjust his/her distance from the herbal steam so that the temperature feels comfortable on the skin of the eyelids.
4. Keep alternating both eyes through the steam for about 10-15 minutes.

NOTE: The distance and the length of time varies with different people but the important key is to *not* burn the skin.

Alternate Method:

1. Make a gauze bag about 5 inches in length and 1.5 inches in width, put in the herbs and sew the bag shut.
2. Fill a pot (like a double boiler) with cold water and put this herbal bag on the top, separated from the water.
3. Steam the bag to warm it.
4. Take the bag out and make sure the temperature is acceptable for the skin of the eyelids.
5. Close the eyelids and rest the bag on the skin for 10 to 15 minutes.

Note: The above information was referenced from the Chinese Medicine Program featured on CCTV 4 on May 1, 2014.

Additional Treatment Approaches

To obtain the quickest and best benefit for the patient, we suggest adding the following self-care methods to his/her herbal treatment.

- The use of artificial lubricant eye drops such as Systane, Refresh, etc. for temporary relief until any eye symptoms subside. Note that a small daily size bottle of lubricant is the best selection since the large size must be used within one month to avoid contamination which could lead to more irritation or even infection.
- The patient can help to relieve symptoms by placing a warm towel or patch over the skin surface of the eyelids for about ten minutes.
- By bathing his/her open eyes in natural sea salt water (made with approximately 1 teaspoon of sea salt) for about 3 to 5 minutes; then rinsing with clean water. NOTE: the salt solution should be easily tolerated so that the patient feels comfortable and does not experience irritation.
- Use herbal patches around the eyes like the Oculax Acupoint Patch for moisturizing the eyes. These patches have also been found to be effective for other eye conditions as well because the herbs move more *blood* and *qi* to the eye in general.

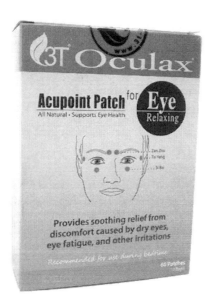

Figure 17 Oculax Acupoint Patches

Diet

The most common cause of dry eye is the normal aging process, especially associated with post-menopausal women. According to TCM classification, these people would have deficiency of liver, kidney and lung *yin* causing too much dryness - not only in the eyes, but also in the mouth, pharynx and throat. Western medicine calls this "Dry Eye Syndrome" or "Sjogren Syndrome". Anyone in this group can use the following herbs to make a tea for preventing *fire* from rising up and causing too much dryness.

To make the tea, take four mugs of water, add the herbs listed in Formula 12 below and cook to three mugs volume. Refrigerate. Each day drink one mug of the tea that has been warmed up on the stove - not in a microwave.

According to traditional Chinese medicine, eating the liver of an animal, especially lamb, is considered to be good for nourishing the eyes. In place of lamb, you can also use beef, pork or chicken liver. However for seniors or persons with high cholesterol, it is better to make a nutritious soup using lean pork rather than lamb. Drink the soup often.

Treatment Principle	Tonify heart *yin*, nourish *blood* and calm the *shen*
Formula 12	Gan Mai Da Zao Tang---Licorice & Jujube Combination[15]
	Gan Cao 15 gm, Xiao Mai or Fu Xiao Mai (undeveloped wheat) - 30 gm, Da Zao - 10 pieces

Treatment Principle	Nourish the liver and moisten the eye
Formula 13	San Zi Yi Ming Tang---Three Seeds Beneficial Vision Soup[16]
	Lean Pork 120 gm, Gou Qi Zi 9gm, Qing Xiang Zi 9 gm, Jue Ming Zi 9 gm
If the patient is weak and has loose bowels but has *yin* deficiency	Remove the Qing Xiang Zi and Jue Ming Zi; use Sha Shen 9 gm, Nu Zhen Zi 9 gm instead

Prevention

Dry eye is due to the aging process and relates more to *yin* deficiency. The key is to keep the body's *yin* and *yang* in balance. Meanwhile, one should avoid environmental issues affecting the overall *yin/yang* balance. Let the eyes rest occasionally when working on the computer or watching television. Also following these activities, a person should warm his/her palms by rubbing the hands together and cup them over the eyes to provide relaxing warmth.

The patient can also make tea using Qi Zi, Mai Dong, Gu Hua, and (with or without) Jue Ming Zi and drink it often.

A practitioner should also be sure to check all of his/her patient's medications for any that have side effects that might be contributing to eye dryness. If this is the case, suggest that the patient contact his/her practitioner prescribing the medication and see if there is an alternate drug available that would not cause dry eyes. Also be aware that if the patient's contact lenses are causing the problem, he/she might need to change those.

References

[1] Soothing Dry Eyes, Health After 50, *The Johns Hopkins Medical Letter*, October, 2007, p. 7

[2] Brochure of the American Academy of Ophthalmology

[3] 針刺治療干眼症的臨床研究, 高衛萍等, 中國針灸, 2004年10月, 第24卷, 第10期, p. 685-687

[4] 逍遙散聯合生脈散治療干眼病的臨床研究, 中國中醫眼科雜誌, 2009年4月, 第19卷, 第2期, p. 71-73

[5] Formula 5: 逍遙散, 中醫眼科學, 廣州中醫學院主編, 上海科學技術出版社, p. 126, #117

[6] Formula 6: 生脈散, Ibid., p. 126, #114

[7] Formula 7: 桑白皮湯, Ibid., p. 124, #52

[8] Formula 8: 杞菊地黃丸, Ibid., p. 123, #34

[9] Formula 9: 增液湯, 現代眼科手冊, 楊鈞主編, 人民衛生出版社, p. 878

[10] Formula 10: 去濕湯, Ibid., p. 876

[11] 八珍湯治療干眼症的臨床觀察, 陳建峰等, 中國中醫眼科雜誌, 2007年6月, 第17卷, 第3期, p. 163-165

[12] Formula 11: 八珍湯, 中醫方劑手冊, 江西中醫學院附屬醫院編, 江西人民出版社, p. 139

[13] Formula 11: 四味湯或稱四君子湯, Ibid., p. 128 + 四物湯, Ibid., p. 134

[14] 中華醫藥, CCTV4 featured on October 3, 2013

[15] Formula 12: 甘麥大棗湯, 中醫方劑手冊, 江西中醫學院附屬醫院編, 江西人民出版社, p. 101

[16] Formula 13: 三子益明湯, 滋補湯水篇, 李南著, p. 101, 香港博益出版集團有限公司

CHAPTER FIVE

Glaucoma

Wǔ Feng Nei Zhang (Five Kinds of *Wind* Cause Internal Obstruction)
Qing Guang Yan (Indigo Light Eye)

Glaucoma includes a group of eye diseases where most - but not all patients - have the symptom of high intraocular pressure (IOP). This high pressure can eventually damage the optic nerve, causing the loss of peripheral vision and ultimately leading to complete blindness.

In the United States and the world, glaucoma is the leading cause of blindness, especially in seniors. According to the National Eye Institute, there were 60.5 million people globally who developed glaucoma in 2010 and that it is likely that only half of the people living with glaucoma are actually aware they have the disease. The reason is that glaucoma initially causes no symptoms, and the subsequent loss of peripheral vision is usually not recognized as being due to this disease.

Causes of Glaucoma

The real cause of glaucoma is still unclear and there is no real cure for it in current medical science. Fortunately, scientists have identified the pathological condition and developed a screening method to detect this disease. As a result patients who have early diagnosis can receive treatment that will control the ongoing damage from the disease to the optic nerve before any vision loss or blindness occurs. Acupuncture and some Chinese herbs can also move the *qi* and *blood* to nourish the eyes to maintain healthier eyes. If acupuncturists work in conjunction with ophthalmologists, this healing combination can slow down the progress of the disease and keep the eye condition from deteriorating. By working together, both TCM and Western medical practitioners can obtain better results than if they worked on their own.

Forms of Glaucoma[1]

There are many forms of glaucoma but the two main types are open-angle and angle-closure. In the United States, the majority of patients have the open-angle form. In contrast, Asians are more likely to have the angle-closure form.

Risk Factors

Strong risk factors for open-angle glaucoma include:

- High intraocular pressure.
- A family history of glaucoma.
- Age 40 years and older for African-Americans; age 60 and older for the general population, especially Mexican-Americans.
- Having a thin cornea.
- Increased cupping of the optic nerve found through ophthalmoscopy exam.

Potential risk factors for open-angle glaucoma include:

- People who have high myopia, diabetes, or hypertension.
- People who have a history of eye surgery or injury, severe anemia, or shock.
- Patients who have used corticosteroids including eye drops, pills, inhalers, and creams.

TCM Observation[2]

Wŭ Feng Nei Zhang is the complete traditional Chinese medical name for glaucoma. The diagnosis is based on the patient's complaints and clinical observation of the color seen when looking through the pupil.

Early TCM doctors observed and used the color seen inside the pupil to describe the different stages of glaucoma. Early onset was diagnosed as *Qing Feng*; *Lu Feng* is the advanced stage; *Huang Feng*, seen more in seniors, is the final stage of complete blindness and may be combined with a fully developed cataract; *Hei Feng* is the same stage as *Huang Feng* but describes a patient without a cataract.

For the past 30 years TCM books have described the colors when seen through the pupil as follows:

- **Indigo:** TCM calls this *Qing Feng Nei Zhang*; onset is slow and without symptoms. This one seems to belong to the open-angle glaucoma form and the majority of it occurs in the United States. As the intraocular pressure (IOP) rises, when you look through the pupil you can see a color change between blue and violet. This is the form of glaucoma that this book focuses on.
- **Green:** TCM identifies this as *Lu Feng Nei Zhang*, with sudden onset and rapid vision loss. This usually belongs to the angle-closure glaucoma form and the majority of this happens to Asians. You will see a green color inside if you look through the pupil.
- **Yellow:** *Huang Feng Nei Zhang* is the advanced stage of glaucoma. When looking through the pupil, there is yellow color inside and the pupil is dilated. There may be a total loss of vision.
- **Black:** TCM identifies *Hei Feng Nei Zhang* as the advanced stage of angle-closure glaucoma. A black color shows inside when seen through the pupil.
- **Dark-Grey or Grey-Red:** *Wū Feng Nei Zhang* is secondary glaucoma. When seen through the pupil, there is a color between black and grey, or grey with red such as smoky fog.

Primary Open-Angle Glaucoma[3]
Qing Feng Nei Zhang

Symptoms

A patient does not have any symptoms in the early course of primary open-angle glaucoma and an examination cannot provide an accurate diagnosis without checking the intraocular pressure (IOP) or the optic disc.

Most of time glaucoma is detected by an optometrist or ophthalmologist during a routine eye exam. Normal reading for the IOP is from 13-15 mm HG although in some cases it can range from 10-21 or even up to 24 mm HG and is still considered acceptable. However, in these latter cases, this type of patient needs his/her IOP rechecked frequently - even up to several times a day. Also if the difference in the reading between both eyes is more than 6 mm HG or if the reading is more than 8 mm HG for the same eye on the same day, the results are diagnostically suspicious.

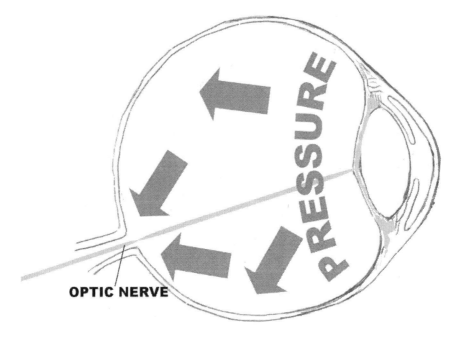

Figure 18 Damage to the Optic Nerve From Increased Pressure of Glaucoma

In Western medicine, besides paying attention to the IOP, early diagnosis can also be made by checking the shape of cupping, color, and the pathways of the blood vessels. In some cases, the patient may have a very high IOP, but does not have any symptoms or changes to the optic nerve so they cannot be diagnosed as glaucoma. Yet in other cases, a patient may have a low IOP, yet both the optic nerve and visual field have been destroyed. This patient is diagnosed with glaucoma.

The primary open-angle glaucoma patient is unaware of having glaucoma until feeling eye discomfort, fatigue, blurred vision, and difficulty seeing at night. The optic nerve can be damaged, causing peripheral vision loss. As the IOP continues to increase, symptoms of eye pain, eyebrow tenderness, and light frontal headaches become evident.

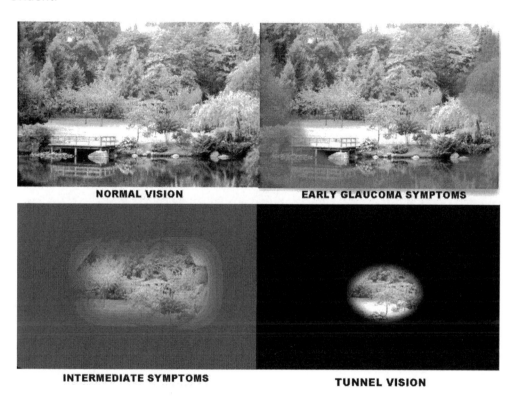

Figure 19 Different Stages of Open-Angle Glaucoma

As the patient's condition worsens, he or she will see a red rainbow-like circle around any light source, experience tunnel vision, and even end up with complete blindness. At this advanced stage, an indigo color is seen behind the pupil. This is a characteristic symptom that is given the Chinese medical name of *Qing Feng Nei Zhang* (Indigo *Wind* Internal Obstruction).

TCM Differential Diagnosis & Treatment[3]

Liver *Qi* Stagnation Transform *Fire*

Symptoms: The patient feels depressed, has painful tension in the eyes and head, fullness in the chest and hypochondrium, fatigue and appetite loss, bitter taste, tongue is red with yellow coat, wiry and fine pulse.

Herbal Treatment

Treatment Principle	Clear *heat*, cool down *fire* and free liver *qi*
Formula 14	Dan Zhi Xiao Yao San---Moutan + Gardenia + Dang Gui & Bupleurum Formula[4]
	(Mu) Dan Pi, Zhi Zi; Chai Hu, Dang Gui, Bai Shao, Fu Ling, Bai Zhu, Gan Cao, Bo He, Sheng Jiang

Liver *Heat* Engender *Wind*

Symptoms: The patient feels tired after work, has discomfort and tension in the eyeballs, foggy mind, emotionally upset or irritable, disturbed sleep, bitter and dry mouth, a red tongue with a yellow coat, and string-like pulse.

Herbal Treatment

Treatment Principle	Clear liver *heat* and extinguish *wind*
Formula 15	Ling Yang Jiao Tang---Antelope Horn Formula[5]
	*Ling Yang Jiao, Ren Shen, Xuan Shen (Hei Shen), Di Gu Pi, Jiang Huo, Che Qian Zi

Phlegm-Fire Harasses the Upper Body

Symptoms: The patient has dizziness and distension in the head, disturbed vision, emotional upset, palpitations, chest oppression, lots of phlegm with nausea, loss of appetite, bitter taste in mouth, red tongue with yellow and greasy coat, string-like, slippery and rapid pulse.

Herbal Treatment

Treatment Principle	Clear liver *heat* and transform *phlegm*, Harmonize the stomach to calm down rebellious *qi*
Formula 16	Huang Lian Wen Dan Tang---Coptis Hoelen and Bamboo Combination[6]
	Huang Lian, #Ban Xia, Chen Pi, Fu Ling, Gan Cao, Zhi Ke, Zhu Ru
For eye pain add	Man Jing Zi, Xia Ku Cao

Yin Deficiency *Wind* Stirring

Symptoms: The patient feels that eye symptoms are worse after work and when feeling tired; there is dizziness and distention in the eyes, blurred vision, he/she sees rainbow circles of light, pupils may be enlarged, insomnia, tinnitus, hot palms, dry mouth, tongue crimson with a slight yellow coat, and a fine pulse.

Herbal Treatment

Treatment Principle	Enrich *yin* and nourish *blood*; soften the liver and extinguish *wind*
Formula 17	E jiao Ji Zi Huang Tang---Donkey Hide with Hen Egg Yolk Formula[7]
	*E jiao, *Ji Zi Huang, Bai Shao, Gou Teng, Sheng Di, Fu Shen, Luo Shi Teng, Shi Jue Ming (abalone shell), Mu Li (oyster shell)

Liver-Kidney Dual Deficiency

Symptoms: This form of the disease is extremely chronic. Vision decreases, the eyeball turns hard, the pupil has enlarged, visual field has narrowed (tunnel vision), the cup of the optic disc is larger and pale when viewed with an ophthalmoscope.

Herbal Treatment

Treatment Principle	Tonify *qi* and *blood* in liver and kidney
Formula 8 For a deficiency of liver-kidney *yin* and *blood*	Qi Ju Di Huang Tang Plus
	Wu Wei Zi, Dang Gui, Bai Shao, Chuan Xiong
Formula 18 Use if the patient is more deficient in kidney *yang* and *essence*	Shen Qi Tang (same name as Fu Gui Di Huang Tang)--- Aconite, Cinnamon + Rehmannia Six Formula[8]
	Plus add on Dang Shen, Huang Qi, Dang Gui, Bai Shao, Chuan Xiong + Tu Si Zi

Acupuncture Treatment

The purpose of acupuncture treatment is to move more *qi* and *blood* to the eye region to nourish the eye and especially the nerve. This keeps the condition stabilized and slows down any deterioration. There was one report where a practitioner selected a single acupuncture point Qiuhou (M-HN-8) for the desired effect of lowering the intraocular pressure (IOP). However, this approach concentrates only on treating the symptoms and will typically just give temporary results. Therefore it is better to select a formula of acupuncture points that will give both temporary relief of the glaucoma symptoms as well as treat the root of the disease in the whole body.

Ocular Needles: Follow the changes observed on the bulbar conjunctiva to select ocuzones. If there are no objective findings, you can choose the Upper (Zone 5), Middle (Zone 8) and Lower Warmer (Zone 13).

Add two or three body points for treatment based on the differential diagnosis. The following are examples of various points to add for different conditions:

1. Liver *qi* stagnation transform *fire* - Hegu (LI 4), Taichong (LR 3), Guangming (GB 37).
2. Liver *heat* engender *wind* - Fengchi (GB20), Neiguan (PC 6), Xingjian (LR 2).
3. Phlegm *fire* harass the upper body - Hegu (LI 4), Neiguan (PC 6), Fenglong (ST 40).
4. *Yin* deficiency *wind* stirring - Shenmen (HT 7), Waiguan (TW 5), Taixi (KI 3), Zulingqi (GB 41).

5. Liver-kidney dual deficiency - Hegu (LI 4), Sanyinjiao (SP 6), Zusanli (ST 36).

Note: The above points are not standard and were selected only as examples. You can switch them and choose other points based on the diagnosis.

Filiform Needles: Choose two to three body points around the eye region; commonly selected are Jingming (BL 1) and Qiuhou (M-HN-8), then add in two to four body points based on the diagnosis.

Seven Star Needles: Five back Shu Points + Geshu (BL 17, associated point of blood), Sanjiaoshu (BL 22, associated point of triple warmer), Qihaishu (BL 24, sea of *qi* hollow, regulates *qi* and *blood*).

There was also one report where an acupuncturist selected the puffy area around Fengchi (GB 20) for needling.[9]

The same report showed that selecting Xinming (see page 85 for more information) had good effect in the treatment of both glaucoma and ARMD. The point is located behind the earlobe and can be found by using an electrical device to find the sensitive area.

Ear Needles: Alternate 3-4 selected points for Eye, Vision 1 or 2, Lung, Heart, Liver, Kidney, and Shenmen.

Moxibustion: Only use for the patient with liver-kidney dual deficiency.

Prevention

Neither Western nor Chinese medical practitioners have yet discovered a way to prevent people from developing glaucoma. However, ophthalmologists from both medical approaches agree that lowering risk is the key to preventing vision loss from this disease. An acupuncturist should work with the patient's ophthalmologist to help control the intraocular pressure.

The key to prevention for glaucoma is a healthy lifestyle that includes regular exercise and a nutritious diet. Details will be introduced in Chapter Eight on Age-Related Macular Degeneration, page 88.

Early Detection: People with high risk factors should have a yearly comprehensive eye exam after the age of 40. After age 60, everyone should have a yearly exam.

One major treatment emphasis of Chinese medicine is for the patient to practice eye exercises and to do self eye massage in order to move *qi* and *blood,* thus enabling better circulation for healthier eyes. Additionally to promote healthy eyes, the patient can take some Chinese herbs based specifically on the character of his/her overall health pattern.

If the patient is not taking any blood thinning medications, he/she can simply take 60 mg of Ginkgo Biloba twice daily for eye health.[10]

Herbal Honey Tea

Treatment Principle	Clear liver *heat*, enrich *yin* nourish liver and brighten the eyes
Formula 19	Qing Guang Ming Shi Tang--- Clear Vision Brighten the Eye[11]
	Gou Qi Zi, Qing Xiang Zi, Sheng Di Huang, Jue Ming Zi (9 mg each) + Bei Sha Shen 15 gm. After boiling, cook on low heat for one hour. Discard the herbs and drink only the tea. Use one cup tea + one tablespoon Honey once a day or twice weekly.

Glaucoma Screening Exams[12]

It is good to understand the glaucoma screening exams listed below:

- **Tonometry:** Measures intraocular pressure (IOP).
- **Visual Field Test:** Measures and documents the entire area seen by the forward-looking eye.
- **Ophthalmoscopy:** Allows the doctor to use an instrument to examine the interior of the eye by looking through the pupil and detecting any damage to the optic nerve caused by glaucoma.

- **Gonioscopy:** Allows the doctor to view the anterior chamber and determine if the iris is closer than normal to the back of the cornea. This test can help diagnose closed-angle glaucoma.
- **Optic Nerve Imaging:** Helps to document any optic nerve changes. Techniques include stereo nerve photographs, scanning laser polarimetry (GDx), and confocal scanning laser ophthalmoscopy (Heidelberg Retinal tomography or HRT).

Secondary Glaucoma

Wū Feng Nei Zhang – "*Wū*" here means the color of dark grey - is not to be confused with the Chinese name for glaucoma (*Wǔ Feng Nei Zhang)* - Five Kinds of Wind Change to Internal Obstruction).

Secondary Glaucoma can be open-angle or closed-angle and have a high intraocular pressure, but the high pressure can be due to some other medical condition in either the eye or body. Because of this, secondary glaucoma often occurs in seniors.

Types of Secondary Glaucoma[1]

1. **Pseudoexfoliation Syndrome:** This occurs when some white material appears to flake off the lens or if the patient has developed a cataract. At some stage of this disease, usually at the intermediate to severe level, the lens excessively extends and pushes into the anterior chamber. This blocks the normal flow of the aqueous humor, resulting in a rise in the IOP. Treatment for this condition is to have surgery as soon as possible.

2. **Neovascular Glaucoma:** Occurs when abnormal vessels grow and block the eye's fluid drainage channels, leading to increased eye pressure. This abnormal growth can be caused by a low blood supply to the eye due to diabetes, insufficient blood flow to the head because of blockage to the cervical artery or its branches, or infarction in the arteries back of the eye.

    Treatment is to perform surgery or undergo medical treatment for the acute symptoms. Herbs can be selected to compliment the treatment for the branch symptoms, but are primarily chosen to treat the root disease that initially caused the glaucoma.

The above two types of secondary glaucoma are caused by mechanical blockages and require surgery as the use of acupuncture and herbal treatments alone would not provide good enough effect.

Another potential cause of glaucoma occurs in seniors who have other health conditions and are taking various types of medications that have a side effect of causing the disease. Therefore it is important for an acupuncturist to know what medications the patient is on and the side effects of those drugs. Drug manufacturers have identified medicines such as corticosteroids and anticholinergic alkaloids like Atropine, etc., that may affect the intraocular pressure. Knowledge of prescription drugs and their side effects will help the acupuncturist better interpret signs and symptoms and to detect disease.

Note that glaucoma is a severe eye disease because the IOP can rise without warning and cause damage to optic nerve resulting in non-reversible vision loss. Although checking the IOP is not in the scope of acupuncture practice, it is okay to touch the eyeball slightly to feel the differing degrees of hardness or softness. If the eyeball feels harder than in a previous visit, the patient should immediately see an ophthalmologist for an IOP exam. Also, the patient should have an IOP exam if a difference in pressure between his/her right and left eyes is found since they should have approximately the same hardness. As a good preventive method, you can teach a patient, who is ready and willing, to regularly touch their eyeballs to feel for the degree of hardness.

References

[1] American Health Assistance Foundation (www.ahaf.org on 2/16/2012)

[2] "青風, 綠風, 黃風內障與閉角型青光眼的辨誤" from 接傳紅等, 中國中醫眼科雜誌 2010年, 第20卷, 第3期, p. 178-180

[3] 中醫眼科學, 廖品正主編, 人民衛出版社, p. 239-252

[4] Formula 14: 丹技逍遙散, 中醫眼科學, 廖品正主編, 人民衛出版社, p. 340, #32

[5] Formula 15: 羚羊角湯, Ibid., p. 347, #175

[6] Formula 16: 黃蓮溫膽湯, Ibid., p. 347, #167

[7] Formula 17: 阿膠雞子黃湯, Ibid., p. 343, #100

[8] Formula 18: 腎氣湯, Ibid., p. 343, #105

[9] "Tapping on the Puffy Area at Fengchi GB 20 and Xinming (new extra point)", from "針灸治療原發性青光眼概況", 遼寧中醫學院附屬醫院, 眼科 赫群, 中國針灸 1999年, 第一期, p. 58-59

[10] "On Protection of Visual Function of Patients with Glaucoma with IOP being controlled" from "銀杏葉制劑對眼壓已控制青光眼患者視功能的保護作用", 林東曉等, 中國中醫眼科雜誌 2005年, 第15卷, 第一期, p. 14-16

[11] Formula 19: 青光明視湯, 李南著, 病後調補湯水篇, 博益出版集團有限公司, Hong Kong, p. 99

[12] Brochure of American Academy of Ophthalmology

CHAPTER SIX

Senile Cataract

Yuan Yi Nei Zhang (Round and Nebulous Internal Obstruction)

The normal process of aging may cause the lens of the eye to go from resilient and transparent to hard and cloudy. This condition, called senile cataract, is the most common type of cataract. It can occur as early as age 40, but is more commonly found in people over the age of 55.

Facts about Cataracts[1]

Cataracts are the leading cause of vision loss in adults 55 and older. According to information from Project ORBIS International, there are about 20 million people blinded because of cataracts, and the number is increasing. In the United States, people do not need to worry too much about going blind from cataracts because of the availability of small incision surgery called phacoemulsification, an advanced microsurgical technique that uses ultrasound to break the cataract apart into small pieces for removal. However in many parts of the world, because of economic underdevelopment, most patients do not have access to this surgery. They might have to wait until a cataract fully develops and blinds them before removal is considered, or they do not have any chance of removal, resulting in a lifetime of blindness.

In Western medicine, the consensus is very clear that there are no medications, eye drops, exercises or eyeglasses that will cause cataracts to disappear or to prevent them from forming in the first place. The only treatment considered is surgery. In sharp contrast, many other types of medical practitioners have reported that early and intermediate stages of cataracts can be treated without surgery. These non-surgical treatments are widely used in China, as well as some other Asian and European countries.

Cataract surgery is big business in United States. Even 20 years ago, there was a report that government and insurance planners had spent more than $3 billion a year towards the cost of cataract care.[2]

On the non-surgical side of cataract treatment, scientists engaged in cataract research are well aware of both the financial savings of using nutritional treatment as well as how it offers an alternative approach if a person is not eligible for surgery. At Tufts' USDA Human Nutrition Research Center on Aging, a leading researcher who has successfully used Vitamins C and E to prevent cataracts remarked, "If you could delay cataract formation by just ten years, you would eliminate the need for half of the cataract extractions". Chinese clinical researchers have come to the same conclusion.

Using sunglasses to reduce the amount of ultraviolet light entering the eyes also reduces the progression of cataracts and macular degeneration.

Cause and Prognosis[3,4]

Senile cataract is related to the aging process and may develop because of changes in the chemical composition of the lens. In Chinese medicine senile cataract is understood to be the result of liver, kidney, or spleen *qi* deficiency. However besides being due to aging, a cataract can also develop from injury - a condition called traumatic cataract. If a cataract develops from certain diseases such as diabetes or from drugs such as corticosteroids, they are called secondary cataracts. If one develops in a newborn baby, the cataract is labeled congenital cataract.

Most of the time, prognosis is good if the patient has a cataract without evidence of any other eye disease. Non-surgical treatment can be used to reverse the early stages of a cataract, as well as to slow down its progression from the intermediate to the advanced stage. If these kinds of treatments are not successful, then surgery is the next option. According to reports by cataract specialist surgeons, the success rate in restoring normal vision by using phacoemulsification combined with intraocular lens (IOL) implant is 98-99%. However, with surgery, there are possible risks and potential complications such as bleeding, infection, swelling or detachment of the retina, glaucoma - any of which can prevent vision from returning to normal as expected.

Symptoms[3,4]

Cataracts usually develop gradually in both eyes without any pain or redness, but can possibly occur only in one eye first. This process can happen so slowly that years may pass before the person notices any reduction in vision. Also, the size and location of the cloudy areas in the lens determines whether a person will be aware that a cataract is developing. If the cataract is located on the cortical layer (outer edge) of the lens, no change in the vision will be noticed for a while. If the cloudiness is located near the nucleus (the center) of the lens, awareness of a problem usually happens faster because the location of the cloudiness interferes with clear vision.

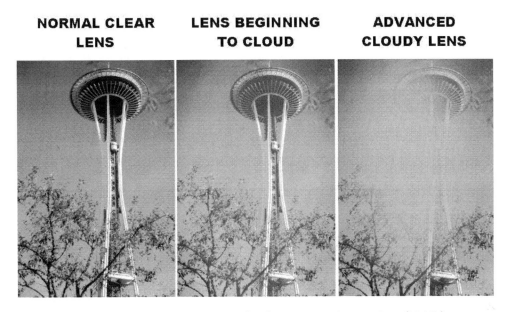

Figure 20 How a Patient Sees Normally (Left), as a Cataract Starts to Form (Middle), and with a Cataract (Right)

In the early stage of a cataract's development, glasses can improve vision. However, over time the glasses become less effective and the patient may frequently change eyeglass prescriptions and yet still experience symptoms that make it more difficult to accomplish daily tasks. Some of these symptoms include:

- Blurred, fuzzy or hazy vision - like looking through a veil.
- Seeing bright colors as dull.
- Having double vision in only one eye.
- An increasing need for more light when reading or doing close work.

- Severe decrease in vision when looking at a bright scene or background.
- Having problems when driving at night with glare, halos or a tail appearing around oncoming car headlights.

If a patient does not treat his/her cataract in time while it ripens or develops, the round-shaped sliver-white or yellowish-dark brown-colored cataract can be observed through the pupil. Blindness and other complications can occur. In the eye exam, this patient can still have HM (hand motion), LP & LR (light perception and reaction), or have LP & LR but cannot see the hand moving. In the early or intermediate stages of a cataract it is difficult to make a clear diagnosis just from the patient's complaints. For a definitive diagnosis, the practitioner needs to use the slit lamp microscope to exam the lens. Also, because the above list of symptoms can result from other diseases besides cataracts, an acupuncturist should suggest that the patient visit an ophthalmologist as soon as possible for a comprehensive medical eye examination, thus allowing the patient to receive early detection of a cataract and/or to exclude other eye diseases.

Learning From a Cataract Case

A man working as a taxi driver felt his vision was getting blurry so he saw an acupuncturist for help and was diagnosed with liver and kidney *yin* deficiency based on TCM differential pattern. He received acupuncture treatment for many months but did not see any improvement in his vision. At this point the acupuncturist referred him to a colleague who prescribed Chinese herbs. However, even after the patient took some of the herbs, he still did not improve and was eventually referred to me (Hoy Ping Chan).

I did not believe these two acupuncturists had checked the patient's vision. They just listened to the patient's complaint and did not really know what his actual visual acuity was. I checked the vision at his first visit, the burred eye that he complained about was 20/200, indicating that he had an advanced cataract. Because he drove a lot for work he required good vision and the cataract needed to be removed as soon as possible. If the previous providers had checked this patient's vision on his first visit, he would not have gone through all those treatments, thus saving him time, money and energy. He should have had surgery as early as possible allowing him to be safer and his work easier.

We can learn three points from this case. First, acupuncturists should have basic Western knowledge of the eye if they treat eye diseases and that acupuncture schools should offer these subjects as part of academic training. Second, when we refer a patient to another practitioner, we should know who the best person is for the referral. Also, if you do not know the Western diagnosis of eye disease, it is hard to know when you should refer. These two acupuncturists had the right diagnosis based on traditional Chinese medicine, but did not have a clear idea which stage of this disease they could help. Third, from this case we should understand how important it is for the integration of East-West medicine. If the patient had come for treatment during the early stages of cataract, TCM treatments could have slowed down the progression of the disease. But because the disease was too advanced, surgery was the best treatment. Both medical approaches have their strengths and weaknesses. The point is that we as practitioners should be able to decide which approach is the better option for giving the patient the best treatment.

TCM Differential Diagnosis and Treatment

The progression of a cataract is chronic and slow. For early and intermediate stages, the best treatment is the use of herbal patent medicines rather than making herbal teas, as patients typically comply better when taking the patents than when cooking and drinking the teas.

Liver-kidney *Essence*, *Qi* and *Blood* Deficiency

Symptoms: Patient has blurred vision, dizziness with tinnitus, low back and knees are sore with weakness, pale face, feeling cold, large volume of clear urine (especially at night), pale tongue with deep-weak pulse.

Herbal Treatment

Deficiency is More of *Qi Essence*

Treatment Principle	Tonify and supplement liver and kidney.
Formula 20	Shi Hu Ye Guang Wan---Dendrobium Combination[5]
	Shi Hu, Sheng Di Huang, Shou Di Huang, Tian Men Dong, Mai Men Dong, Ren Shen, Shan Yao, Tu Si Zi, Gou Qi Zi, Rou Cong Rong, Fu Ling, Gan Cao, Cao Jue Ming, Ju Hua, Bai Ji Li, Qing Xiang Zi, Fang Feng, *Ling Yang Jiao, *Xi Jiao, Chuan Xiong, Chuan Lian, Niu Xi, Zhi Ke, Xing Ren, Wu Wei Zi

Deficiency is More of Liver-Kidney *Yin*

Treatment Principle	Enrich and nourish liver and kidney *yin*
Formula 8	Qi Ju Di Huang Wan

Deficiency is More of Kidney *Yang*

Treatment Principle	Tonify and supplement kidney *yang*
Formula 21	You Gui Wan---Eucommia & Rehmannia Formula[6]
	Shou Di, Shan Zhu Yu, Shan Yao, Dang Gui, Rou Gui, Gou Qi, *Lu Jiao Jiao, Tu Si Zi, Zhi Fu Zi, Du Zhong

Deficiency and Weakness of Spleen *Qi*

Treatment Principle	Fortify and boost spleen *yang*
Formula 1	Bu Zhong Yi Qi Wan

Deficiency of *Blood* and *Liver Fire* Flames Upward

Treatment Principle	Enrich *yin* and bring down the *fire* and enrich *blood* to brighten the eye
Formula 22	Yi Yin Shen Qi Wan---Benefit the Kidney *Yin* and *Qi* Pill[7] + Zhen Zhu Mu (Pearl Powder)
	Fu Ling, Ze xie, Dang Gui Wei, Dan Pi, Wu Wei Zi, Shan Zhu Yu, Chai Hu, Shou Di Huang, Sheng Di Huang, Chen Sha

Acupuncture Treatment

A patient will obtain the most benefit by receiving a series of 6-10 acupuncture treatments once or twice a year. The acupuncturist uses points around the eye in addition to choosing one or two body points such as Zusanli (ST 36), Sanyinjiao (SP 6), Taichong (LV 3), Taixi (KI 3), and Yongquan (KI 1) to strengthen the vision.

Seven Star Needle: Tapping on Ganshu (BL 18), Pishu (BL 20), Shenshu (BL 23) can increase treatment effectiveness when combined with local eye point needling.

The patient will also benefit if the acupuncturist teaches him/her to put Oculax herbal patches around the eye points at night as shown below:

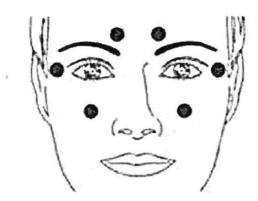

Figure 21 Placement of Oculax Herbal Eye Patches

Moxibustion may be effective by using walnut shell or *lei huo jiu* (moxa stick) to promote *qi* and *blood* to the eyes. For details, refer to the ARMD chapter, page 86.

Self-Massage: Suggest to the patient that he/she does self-massage around both eyes and on both ears. Rub until the ears feel warm to the touch, then follow the warm up with emphasis on the auricular points for Eye, Liver and Kidney.

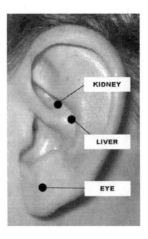

Figure 22 Self-massage Points for Treating Cataracts

Dietary and Other Treatments

Treatment Principle	Support nutrition and brighten the eye
Formula 23 Herbal soup formula from Lui Hui Ying, herbal medicine eye doctor	Man Jing Zi powders[8] (5 gm) + Pork (50 gm)
	Cook in a double boiler, adding enough water to cover the ingredients. Boil until the meat is done (usually takes more than one hour). Eat the soup often.

Supplements[2]

- Gary Price Todd, M.D., ophthalmologist and author of *Nutrition, Health and Disease*, suggests doing a hair lab analysis first, then to attempt to balance the patient's mineral levels by supplementing with those minerals in which he/she is deficient. Most people are found to be lacking in zinc, while some are found deficient in copper, manganese, or selenium. Dr. Todd would also supplement with certain vitamins including beta-carotene, B complex and E vitamins, Bioflavonoids and the enzyme glutathione.

- Stuart Kemeny, M.D. an eye, ear, nose and throat specialist whose training included optometry and ophthalmology, has treated 7,000 cataract patients with a nutrition program that was modeled on European practices. In his book *Cataract Breakthrough*, he recommends a daily vitamin intake of Vitamin C with bioflavonoids 500 mg 2 or 3 times daily with meals, Vitamin E 400 IUs 2 or 3 times daily (note that people with high blood pressure should not exceed 400 IU a day), selenium 100 mg twice daily, Vitamin A with Zinc 30,000 unit once daily, Vitamin B Complex 100 mg once daily taken after breakfast (note that people with cancer should omit the B complex).

EYE DROPS

Treatment Principle	Clear the eyesight
Formula 24	Xie Zhu Ming Mu Ye---Musk and Pearl Eyedrops[9]
	*Xie Xiang (dry grains or powders are the secretion from the male organ of deer) + *Zhen Zhu (pearl powders)

Formula 25	ZYM Di Yan Ye[10]
	Ma Fan Shi Eye Drops (made from igneous rocks of a volcano)

A commercially available eye drop formula from Switzerland is *Jing Ling* (Vitreolent Eye Drops), made of Potassium Iodide 3mg and Sodium Iodide 3mg.

Prevention

For healthy eyes, as with other eye diseases, people should have a healthy life-style, eat a balanced diet and protect their eyes from ultraviolet light. Since cataract development is related to the liver, kidney and spleen *qi*, *yin* and *yang* balance, maintain it by alternating the common herbal formulas such as the following:

Treatment Principle	Tonify liver and kidney *yin*
Formula 26	Liu Wei Di Huang Wan---Rehmannia Six Formula[11]
	Fu Ling, Mu Dan Pi, Shan Yao, Shan Zhu Yu, Shou Di Huang, Ze Xie

Treatment Principle	Tonify kidney *yang*
Formula 27	Bu Shen Wan (also named Tu Si Zi Wan)---Cuscutae Semen Pill[12]
	Tu Si Zi, Ze Xie, Xi Xin, Wu Wei Zi, Chong Wei Zi, Shan Yao, Shou Di Huang

Treatment Principle	Tonify kidney *yin, yang* and *blood*
Formula 28	Wu Zi Tea---Five Seed Tea
	Gou Qi Zi (Lycium fruit), Tu Si Zi (Cuscuta), Sang Shen Zi (Muberry), Che Qian Zi (Plantago Seed), Nu Zhen Zi (Ligustrum)

To Make Wu Zi Tea

In this formula, the first three seeds - Gou Qi Zi (Lycium fruit), Tu Si Zi (Cuscuta), and Sang Shen Zi (Muberry) are the base, functioning to tonify *yin, yang* and *blood*.

The 4th and 5th seeds in the formula, Che Qian Zi (Plantago Seed) and Nu Zhen Zi (Ligustrum) are used to specifically treat the patient's condition. Alternative seeds to choose from according to a patient's condition can be found in the following list:

- Che Qian Zi for clearing *heat*, promoting diuresis, and clearing eyesight (visual acuity).

- Nu Zhen Zi for tonifying the liver and kidney *yin*, promoting eyesight, helping dizziness and tinnitus, and helping graying hair change back to its original color.
- Wu Wei Zi for tonifying *qi* and liver function. This herb helps fatigue and people with vertigo due to Meniere's disease, and can also help people sleep. It is not indicated if the patient is constipated.
- Jue Ming Zi for suppressing liver *yang* and clearing liver *heat–fire*, clearing eyesight, and helping to improve bowel function. If the patient has loose bowels or diarrhea, do not use this seed. This herb can also help control high lipid levels. Refer to page 90 and 110 for the formula.
- Lian Zi for tonifying spleen *qi*, relieving diarrhea, benefiting kidney *essence*, nourishing heart *yin*.
- Qing Xiang Zi for clearing liver *heat-fire*, removing the nebula (the opacity of the cornea) and clearing eyesight, calming liver *yang*.
- Jin Ying Zi for reducing frequent urination, relieving nocturnal emission, and tonifying kidney *yang*.
- Fu Pen Zi for tonifying the liver and kidney *qi*, promoting eyesight and preserving kidney *essence*.
- Di Fu Zi for clearing *heat* and as a diuretic, benefiting skin problems, alleviating itching.
- Man Jing Zi for easing and expelling the *wind-heat* on the eye and head, benefitting eyesight, helping conjunctivitis, and *wind-heat* types of headache and cold.

For keeping eyes healthy, anyone can also use Dr. Gary P. Todd's Basic Prevention Formula: Vitamin C 1200 mg, Vitamin E 400 I.U., and Zinc 20 mg.

For people with diabetes there is an article[13] written by Li Rui and Jin Ming, that points out the relationship between diabetes and the development of cataracts. The research showed that oxidative damage plays an important role in the pathogenesis of a diabetic cataract and that there are several micronutrients that help to prevent a cataract from progressing. These are the groups of antioxidant vitamins such as A, B-complex, C, E, and enzymes from the metal elements of zinc, magnesium, selenium, chromium, iron, and copper. Supplements specifically made for eye health such as

I-Cap and Ocuvite are available over-the-counter. Taking the appropriate amount of these micronutrients can delay the development of cataracts.

We would also like to introduce a simple, non-Chinese treatment method because it is easy to try and does not seem to have any harmful side effects. The suggestion is to take 1000 mg of bilberry daily. Bilberry has been used in European societies for centuries and modern research confirms its active constituent is anthocyanosides, a type of bioflavonoid that nutritionally supports blood flow throughout the body, especially in the tiny capillaries that flow to the eyes.

The best overall preventive measure is for the senior to have a comprehensive medical eye exam that can provide early diagnosis for any senior eye condition, thus helping him/her to choose the right treatment to protect against vision loss.

References

[1] KRAMES Communications Booklet

[2] Chapter 9, Cataract Surgery – Another Unnecessary Operation? In the book *What Your Doctor Won't Tell You*; Gary Price Todd, M.D.'s Formula and Stuart Kemeny's Formula

[3] Brochure of American Academy of Ophthalmology

[4] Brochure of American Health Assistance Foundation

[5] Formula 20: 石斛夜光丸, 中醫眼科學, 廖品正主編, 人民衛生出版社, p. 340, #43

[6] Formula 21: 右歸丸, Ibid., p. 340, #46

[7] Formula 22: 益陰腎氣丸, 現代眼科手冊, 楊鈞主編, 人民衛生出版社, p. 876

[8] Formula 23: 蔓荊子湯, "老年白內障中醫治療現狀" 高延娥等, 甘肅中醫, 2003年, 第16卷, 第5期, p. 15

[9] Formula24: 麝珠明目液, Ibid.

[10] Formula 25: 麥飯石滴眼液, Ibid.

[11] Formula 26, 六味地黃丸, 中醫眼科學, 廖品正主編, 人民衛生出版社, p. 340, #36

[12] Formula 27: 補腎丸 (又名菟絲子丸), Ibid. p. 343, # 97

[13] "微量營養素與糖尿病性白內障", 李蕊, 金明, 中國中醫眼科雜誌, 2009年, 第19卷, 第1期, p. 55

CHAPTER SEVEN

Vitreous Humor Diseases

Yun Mu Yi Jing (Cloud and Fog Move into the Eye)
Zhu Zhong Dong Qi (*Qi* Is Moving Inside the Eye)
Shi Zhan Hun Miao (Blurred Vision as Mist)
Shi Zhan You Se (Blurred Vision as Seen Color in the Eye)

The vitreous humor is a nearly transparent gel composed of approximately 99% water, hyaluronic acid acting as a lubricant, and collagen fibers for support. There are no blood vessels in the vitreous humor - its nutrition comes from the aqueous humor and choroid. The gel fills in the vitreous chamber to support the retina and to hold the shape of the eyeball, even protecting against a strike to the retina and eyeball. Another of its important functions for vision is refraction.[1] Because the metabolism of the vitreous humor is very slow, if there are any changes to its flow of nutrients the vitreous gel will not be replaced. Western medicine has created a substance to use as a substitute but it does not work as well as natural vitreous.

Chinese medicine calls the pupil *tong shen* and the vitreous *shen gao* (god's gel), and relates them to the Water Wheel. This location is the same source as the kidney and liver so diseases in *shen gao* are considered to be from an imbalance of liver-kidney functions.

Floaters (Degeneration of the Vitreous)[2]

Many seniors see small dots, lines, clouds, or cobwebs that move across the visual field from time to time. These objects are most visible when looking at a plain surface, such as a blue sky or a white wall. Although they appear to be in front of the eye, they are actually floating in the vitreous humor. This phenomenon is caused by shadows cast on the retina from microscopic structures within the vitreous body. As we age, the vitreous humor gradually begins to liquefy, its supportive fibers dissolve, condense and contract to form these various sizes and shapes of microscopic structures called floaters.

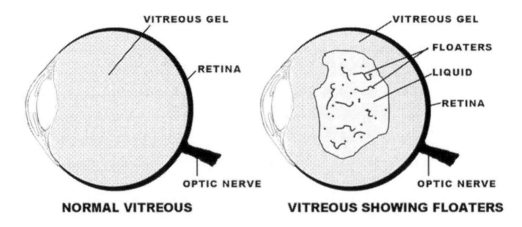

Figure 23 Normal Vitreous (L) and Vitreous with Floaters (R)

These floaters, a result of the normal aging process, usually do not need treatment because they do not cause vision loss, although they can sometimes be annoying.

Most often floaters occur in both eyes but if a patient has previously had localized eye disease, the debris will usually be found only in the previously affected eye. Other kinds of health conditions or injury that cause bleeding from other parts of the eye can cause floaters to affect just one eye.

TCM Differential Diagnosis and Treatment[3,4]

The development of floaters relates to liver-kidney deficiency. As a result of aging, kidney and liver function weaken causing deficiency of *essence*, *qi* and *blood* and make them unable to ascend enough to nourish the eye. Thus the vitreous humor degenerates and the floaters occur.

Symptoms: Some patients describe the symptoms to be like a mosquito flying in front of the eye, so floaters are also called *Fei Wen Zheng (*Mosquito Flying Symptom*)*. Floaters may stay the same for years without much change. If this symptom appears in a young or middle-aged person without any other physical changes in the body, it is a physiological condition with no need for treatment. But if floaters occur in a senior, a comprehensive medical eye examination is needed to exclude other eye diseases before treating the patient with Chinese medicine. If the patient notices a sudden shower of floaters, persistent flashing lights in one eye, or a partial blockage in his/her vision field, it is important to have an immediate evaluation to determine if there is a retinal tear or if a retinal detachment has occurred. No treatment should be given before a definitive diagnosis has been made.

Eye disease treatment in Chinese medicine emphasizes addressing the root disorder causing the disease. Thus if the floaters do not cause any vision problems, treatment might not be necessary as they represent a branch, not the root, of the problem. But most of the time seniors usually already have disorders in the *zang-fu*. If the practitioner does not pay attention to these conditions, this patient may not just have floaters, but other illnesses that might appear later on.

The four kinds of *zang-fu* imbalance that can cause floaters are discussed below.

Liver-Kidney *Yin* Deficiency

Herbal Treatment

Treatment Principle	Tonify liver and kidney *yin*
Formula 29 Based on the patient's health condition choose Ming Mu Di Huang Wan or Qi Ju Di Huang Wan or Zhi Bai Di Huang Wan or Zi Shen Ming Mu Wan	Ming Mu Di Huang Wan---Rehmannia Eye Bright Pills[5]
	Shu Di Huang, Shan Yao, Shan Zhu Yu, Mu Dan Pi, Ze Xie, Fu Ling + Shi Jue Ming, Bai Shao, Bai Ji Li, Dang Gui, Ju Hua, Gou Qi Zi

Qi and *Blood* Dual Deficiency

Symptoms: Appear after major surgery, long term internal illness or malnutrition due to being on a diet; the patient shows fatigue, shortness of breath, general weakness with pale lips and tongue, and a fine pulse.

Herbal Treatment

Treatment Principle	Supplement both *qi* and *blood*; enrich liver and kidney function
Formula 30 or use **Formula 11**, Ba Zhen Tang	Shi Quan Da Bu Wan---Ginseng and Angelica Ten Combination Pill[6]
	Dang Shen, Bai Zhu, Fu Ling, Zhi Gan Cao, Dang Gui, Chuan Xiong, Shou Di Huang, Bai Shao, Huang Qi, Rou Gui

For the patient with a mild condition, it is good to alternate the above two formulas (Shi Quan Da Bu Wan and Ba Zhen Tang). However, if the patient needs long term treatment it is suggested that he/she takes the *wan* formula instead of the *tang*. Also, if the patient's overall condition is more severe, you should first use *tang*; then switch to using *wan* after the patient's condition stabilizes.

In both the Liver-Kidney *Qi* Deficiency and *Qi-Blood* Dual Deficiency types, floaters usually appear in both eyes.

Spleen *Qi* Deficiency with Internal *Dampness* and *Heat*

Symptoms: The spleen *yang* is disturbed, the body shows middle burner *damp heat* gathering in the gallbladder, blocking the liver *qi* from moving upward to affect the eye causing floaters.

Herbal Treatment

Treatment Principle	Dispel the *dampness* and clear the *heat*
Formula 31	Wen Dan Tang---Bamboo & Hoelen Combination[7]
	#Ban Xia, Chen Pi, Fu Ling, Gan Cao, Zhi Shi, Zhu Ru

Liver *Fire* Flaming Upward, Frenetic Movement of *Hot Blood*

Symptoms: Emotional disturbance causes ascendant hyperactivity of liver *yang*, with the result that *fire* flames upward causing blood to leak into the vitreous. Note that there are no blood vessels in the vitreous. If blood does leak into the vitreous it can range from a very little amount or accumulate enough to block vision. In this latter case, you can see red color throughout the pupil which means that there is blood in the vitreous chamber - a very severe condition. In this case, you should immediately send the patient to an ophthalmologist for evaluation because in Western medicine this is no longer diagnosed as floaters. Also before any treatment, you must know if the blood in the vitreous chamber is new bleeding or has been there for some time - indicating it had already stopped - because the treatment principles are different. It will make the condition worse if you choose the wrong formula.

Herbal Treatment For Fresh Bleeding

Treatment Principle	Cool and stanch *blood*
Formula 32 **Note:** *DO NOT* do acupuncture if there is fresh bleeding	Ling Xue Tang---Staunch the Bleeding Combination[8]
	Xian He Cao, Han Lian Cao, Sheng Di Huang, Zhi Zi Tan, Bai Shao, Bai Ji, Bai Lian, Ce Bai Ye, *E Jiao, Bai Mao Gen

Herbal Treatment For *Blood* Stasis

Treatment Principle	Quicken the *blood* and dispel stasis
Formula 33	Tao Hong Si Wu Tang---Persica and Carthamus Four Herb Combination[9]
	Sheng Di Huang, Chi Shao, Chuan Xiong, Dang Gui Wei, Tao Ren, Hong Hua
plus add in **Formula 34**	Er Chen Tang---Citrus & Pinellia Combination[10]
	#Ban Xia, Chen Pi, Fu Ling, Gan Cao

Acupuncture Treatment

Use the cataract protocol for treating floaters and stagnant *blood* in the vitreous chamber. Remember: do not do acupuncture if the vitreous chamber has fresh bleeding.

Prevention

Prevention for vitreous health is also the same as for cataract: people should have a healthy lifestyle and eat a balanced diet. There is a correlation between vitreous health and a balance of *qi, yin* and *yang* of the spleen, liver and kidney. For an effective herbal patch for vitreous problems and helpful herbal formulas (#23, 26, 27 and 28), refer to Chapter Six, pages 64-66.

References

[1] " Is It a Floater---or a Detached Retina?", *The Johns Hopkins Medical Letter---Health After 50*, Volume 13, Issue 8, October 2001, p. 4-5

[2] Group Health Tri-region Eye Service and the Center for Health Promotion Pamphlet Service

[3] 現代眼科手冊, 楊鈞主編, 人民衛生出版社, p. 856

[4] 眼科中醫學, 廣州中醫學院主編, 上海科學技術出版社, p. 83

[5] Formula 29: 明目地黃丸, Ibid., p. 126, #122

[6] Formula 30: 十全大補丸, Ibid., p. 123, #28

[7] Formula 31: 溫膽湯, Ibid., p. 125, #96

[8] Formula 32: 寧血湯, Ibid., p.126, #111

[9] Formula 33: 桃紅四物湯, Ibid., p.124, #59

[10] Formula 34: 二陳湯, Ibid., p. 122, #7

CHAPTER EIGHT

Age-Related Macular Degeneration
(AMD or ARMD or SMD)

Shi Zhan Hun Miao (Blurred Vision as Mist)
Shi Wu Bian Xing (Distorted Vision)
Shi Zhan You Se (Blurred Vision as Seen Color in the Eye)
Bao Mang (Sudden Blindness)

ARMD is a dangerous eye disorder which is the leading cause of severe vision loss among people older than sixty-five. More than 13 million Americans have early signs of this disease, and about two million have progressed to the point of visual impairment - about 5% of seniors.

Facts About ARMD

Macular Degeneration causes deterioration of the macula and damages the central vision. The macula is the heart of the eye's vision center and is responsible for sharp and high-definition vision to manage reading, writing, recognizing faces, driving, and to distinguish fine details and color. The true underlying cause of ARMD is still unclear so there is only limited treatment available for these patients to help control the disease, but not to cure it.[1,2,3]

Risk Factors[1,2,3]

The causes of ARMD are not well understood, but researchers have analyzed what major risk factors can increase the possibility of developing the disease. The following is a list of these factors:

- **Aging:** The risk increases with age. People in their 50's have a 2% chance of developing ARMD. People between the ages of 64 and 74 have a 25% chance. People 75 years or older have more than a 30% chance.
- **Gender:** More ARMD patients are female.
- **Genetics:** A family history of this disease increases the risk.
- **Race:** In the United States, Caucasians and people with light-colored eyes have increased risk.
- **Habits:** Cigarette smokers or people who have smoked in the past 15 years have more than double the chance of getting the disease.
- **Diet:** People with a lower consumption of fruits and vegetables are more susceptible.
- **Bright Sunlight:** People without good sunglass protection who were exposed directly to bright sunlight or ultraviolet radiation at a young age.
- **Supplement Deficiency:** Antioxidant Vitamins C and E, the mineral zinc, carotenoids, lutein and zeaxanthin.
- **Health Conditions:** People with hypertension, high cholesterol, coronary artery disease, diabetes, obesity and hyperopia; also some researchers think that cataract surgery may be connected to an increased risk of ARMD.
- **Inactivity:** Exercise improves cardiovascular health, moves more blood to the eye to support the cells in the macula preventing deterioration.

Symptoms[1,2,3]

In the early stages of ARMD, a patient usually does not have any complaints about his or her eyes. Many seniors can already have macular degeneration and be totally unaware of it, especially if the disease only affects one eye.

In Western medicine, the diagnosis of ARMD is has two categories, the dry form and wet form.

- Dry ARMD: Also called atrophic or non-neovascular, affects the vast majority - about 90% - of patients with ARMD. The progression of this form is very slow. As time passes, the patient may complain of having blurred vision and gradually start to experience difficulty with reading, writing and distinguishing faces. As the condition advances, the patient may complain about difficulties with driving and seeing a blind spot at the center of the visual field. Eyesight is hindered as the spot gets larger. It is important to know that the dry form can suddenly change to the wet form without any warning signs. A patient must self-monitor his/her vision daily by using the Amsler Grid test. Details are given on pages 91-92.

AMSLER GRID TEST

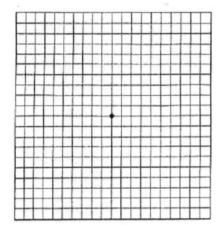
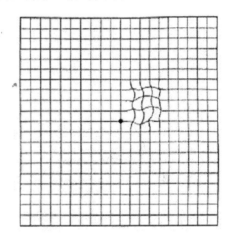

NORMAL VISION   **EARLY ARMD**

Figure 24 Amsler Grid Test Showing Normal (L) and Early ARMD (R) Results

- Wet ARMD: This is also called exudative or neovascular ARMD. The earliest sign of this wet form is that the patient has distorted vision caused by the growth in the choroid of new abnormal blood vessels called choroidal neovascularization (CNV). These abnormal blood vessels first leak fluid, then blood, under the macula. A faded color might appear and a blind spot can develop in the macula, the center of the focusing area. Unless this fluid or blood is absorbed, it can possibly cause the formation of scar tissue and eventually lead to a partial loss of central vision.

Overall, the progression of ARMD may end in legal blindness because of extreme damage to the central vision. However it does not affect the peripheral vision and does not lead to complete blindness. In this advanced stage ARMD patients have a unique way of walking because they cannot see what is straight ahead of them. They have to move their head left and right in order to use their peripheral vision. If you see a patient walking this way it should immediately make you suspicious that he/she may be an ARMD patient.

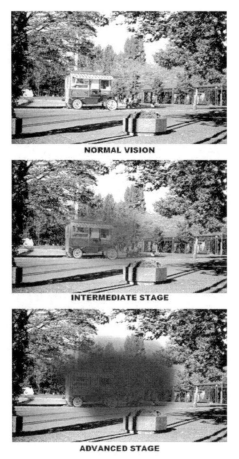

Figure 25 Progression of Macular Degeneration as seen by the Patient

The Structure and Pathophysiology of ARMD[1]

The Retina: This is the paper thin tissue lining the back of the eye. Containing ten layers of tissue, the retina has two kinds of visual cells called cones and rods. Located at the center of the retina, the macula has funnel-shaped side walls with cells arranged in special order, and a very small deep dent at its center named the fovea centralis (foveola). This tiny thin tent is both an avascular zone and also a rod-free area, containing the visual cells holding only the cones. They are most sensitive to light and allow sharp straight-ahead vision by sending visual signals to the brain. The cones respond to bright color vision and enable the recognition of details of shapes. The rods work for dim light vision. This is the reason that patients with severe macular degeneration are counted as legally blind.

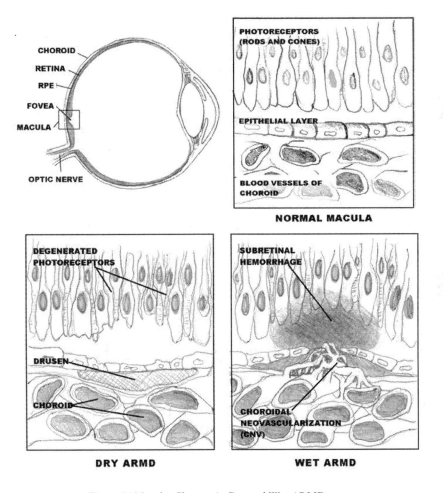

Figure 26 Macular Changes in Dry and Wet ARMD

RPE Layer: This is retinal pigment epithelium located at the outermost layer of the retina. It contains very active cells that provide power for absorbing light and supporting the function of visual cells. The cells of RPE have colors due to melanin and lipofuscin. When observed through the ophthalmoscope, a patient in the earliest stage of ARMD has some yellow deposits called drusen that form beneath the retina. Drusen deposits are thought to be produced from the metabolic waste of the RPE layer. In the beginning, these deposits usually do not affect vision. However, when drusen expands in size and quantity, the retina gets thinner and causes the cones to decay up to the point that they die. Ultimately this causes the central vision to gradually decrease, leading to severe loss of eyesight. This condition is categorized as the dry form of ARMD.

A second function of the RPE is to protect and nourish the retina. Its exterior connects the Bruch's membrane providing support to the retina as well as separation from the choroid, considered to be the 'blood bank' of the retina.

In the wet form of ARMD, abnormal blood vessels growing underneath the macula are very fragile and can leak fluid or blood into the macula, resulting in sudden, severe vision loss.

TCM Relationship Between the Macula and Organs[4,5]

Chinese medical scientists consider the macula to have a very close relationship to the Five Organs. The occurrence of ARMD relates to the malfunction of the kidney, spleen and/or liver.

- Kidney is the root of the congenital essential substance, responsible for growth and development. According to the Five Wheels Theory of the eye, the pupil belongs to the kidney, and because the macula is located on the same straight line from the pupil to the back of the eye, it is counted as belonging to the kidney as well. The *original essence* stored in the kidneys is rich and strong, resulting in eyesight that is clear and bright. The occurrence of ARMD relates to the weakness of the kidney function during the aging process. The kidney is said to be the "house of *water* and *fire*", where the kidney *yin* and *yang* both restrict and promote each other in the human body to maintain balance. If either one fails, it creates an imbalance between the *yin* and *yang*, which can manifest as *water* insufficiency or *fire* excess. These conditions are the causes of blurred vision and other eye problems.

- **Spleen-Stomach** is the acquired root and the source of production and nutrition. Using the six-channel pattern identification system, Dr. Wang Ming Fong considers that the spleen manages the color yellow, so the macula belongs to the foot Taiyin Spleen channel. Thus the occurrence of macular degeneration can relate to spleen malfunction of transportation and transformation. Ancient TCM considers that the center of a piece of land belongs to the spleen, and since the macula is located at the center of the retina, the macula belongs to spleen as well. Deficiency of the spleen *qi* causes blurred vision.
- **Liver** is the *sea of blood* and one of its functions is the storage of *blood*. Both liver and kidney are derived from the same source, so the *blood* and *essence* grow mutually. The macula connects to the choroid which is full of blood from the liver, receiving rich nutrition to maintain bright and clear eyesight. The liver's point of entry is the eye. Because the Liver channel goes up to connect to the eye, it is the main organ affecting vision. Deficiency of liver *yin* may lead to blurred vision and other eye problems. When liver *qi* is balanced, *qi* flows freely and reflects a state of harmony. Stagnation of liver *qi* causes the eye to have difficulty discerning color and can even lead to sudden blindness.

In conclusion, as people age their kidney and liver *qi* decrease naturally and the spleen *qi* sinks, causing drusen to develop in the macula. This early stage is a deficiency pattern. As the pattern continues, the pathological condition changes from deficiency to *dampness, phlegm* and *blood* stagnation. The function of the organs no longer works normally causing the *essence* and the *blood* to leak out from the vessels, resulting in severe vision loss.

This advanced stage of ARMD is an excess pattern. It starts with deficiency at the root and progresses to excess in its branch, ultimately becoming a mixture of both deficiency and excess patterns.

TCM Differential Diagnosis and Treatment[4,5]

Liver-Kidney Deficiency

Symptoms: These may occur in the dry form, the early stage of wet form, or if a scar has developed. The patient experiences blurred vision with a dim spot in front of his/her eyes and the eyes feel dry; there is dizziness, tinnitus, weakness and soreness of the back and knees. Other symptoms include sleeplessness with lots of dreams, a red tongue with thin coating and a fine pulse.

Herbal Treatment

Treatment Principle	Supplement liver and kidney *yin* and dispel stasis
Formula 35	Si Wu Tang + Wu Zi Wan---Angelica Four and Five Seed Combination[6]
	Dang Gui, Shou Di Huang, Bai Shao, Chuan Xiong + Gou Qi Zi, Tu Si Zi, Wu Wei Zi, Di Fu Zi, Che Qian Zi

Acupuncture Treatment

Ocular Needles: Ocuzones Kidney (Zone 3), Upper Warmer (Zone 5), Liver (Zone 6); or choose other zones that exhibit changes.

Use these ocuzone points in conjunction with:

Baihui (GV 20), Xingjian (LR 2), Taixi (KI 3).

Filiform Needles: Qiuhou (M-HN-8), Taiyang (M-NH-9), Hegu (LI 4), Xingjian (LR 2), Taixi (KI 3).

Seven Star Needle: Five Back Shu Points of Feishu (BL 13), Xinshu (BL 15), Ganshu (BL 18), Pishu (BL 20), Shenshu (BL 23).

Ear Needles: Ear points for Eye, Liver, Kidney, Spleen, Shenmen.

Scalp Needle: #18 below the occipital line.

Spleen *Qi* Deficiency

Symptoms: These may occur in both dry and wet forms. Symptoms include blurred and distorted vision; viewing through an ophthalmoscope shows faded color change and exudation of fluid or blood under the macula. The patient has fatigued eyes often leading to closed eyelids, weakness in the body and a foggy mind, the tongue is pale with white coating and a weak pulse.

Herbal Treatment

Treatment Principle	Tonify spleen *yang* and spleen *qi*
Formula 1 Plus and Minus For dry type	Bu Zhong Yi Qi Tang - Plus and Minus
	Huang Qi, Dang Shen, Dang Gui, Chen Pi, Chai Hu, Bai Zhu, Sheng Ma, Ge Gen, Dan Shen, *Di Long, Fu Ling, Mi Meng Hua,
For wet type add	San Qi, Bai Mao Gen; #Xi Cao Gen

Acupuncture Treatment

Wait for any bleeding to stop before using acupuncture.

Ocular Needles: Ocuzones Upper Warmer (Zone 5), Middle Warmer (Zone 8), Spleen (Zone 11); or choose other zones with observed changes.

Add in body points: Baihui (GV 20), Taiyuan (LU 9), Sanyinjiao (SP 6).

Filiform Needles: Yangbai (GB 14), Sibai (ST 2), Taiyang (M-HN-9); or Lieque (LU 7), Sanyinjiao (SP 6); or Qihai (CO 6), Xuehai (SP 10), Fenglong (ST 40).

Seven Star Needle: Upper Five Back Shu Point + Geshu (BL 17).

Moxibustion: Yinbai (SP 1); or Xuehai (SP 10).

Yin Deficiency *Fire* Intensity

Symptoms: Note that these symptoms can appear suddenly without warning. They include vision loss and distortion which can change to severe vision loss in a short time; dry mouth, night sweats, lot of dreams, red tongue with thin coating. Ophthalmoscopic examination shows fresh blood on the macula.

Herbal Treatment

Treatment Principle	Enrich *yin* and descend *fire*; cool and stanch the bleeding
Formula 36	Zhi Bai Di Huang Tang Plus and Minus---Anemarrhena, Phellodendron & Rehmannia Formula[7]
	Zhi Mu, Sheng Di Huang, Mu Dan Pi, Ze Xie; Xuan Shen, Chi Shao, Han Lian Cao, Bai Mao Gen, Zhi Zi Tan, Che Qian Zi, San Qi, *Di Long

Phlegm-Dampness Internal Gathering

Symptoms: Include vision loss, distorted vision, lots of drusen seen with an ophthalmoscope, disorderly pigment cells, along with exudation pooling into different sizes of spots. The patient may feel chest oppression, have poor appetite and sluggish digestion, thirst with no desire to drink, red tongue with a yellow greasy coat, string-like and slippery pulse.

Herbal Treatment

Treatment Principle	Dispel *dampness* and expel *phlegm*, clear *heat* to brighten the eye
Formula 37	San Ren Tang Plus and Minus---Triple Nut Combination[8]
	Xing Ren, Bai Kou Ren, Yi Yi Ren; Hua Shi, #Ban Xia, Hou Po, Tong Cao, Dan Zhu Ye
For severe *heat* pattern add	Zhi Zi, Huang Qin, Long Dan Cao

Phlegm-Stasis Accumulation

Symptoms: Vision loss, distorted vision, a dim red tongue with stasis speckles and thin coat, deep and rough pulse. Ophthalmoscopic exam shows macular area color changes to a bruised or crimson color and *blood* stagnation.

Herbal Treatment

Treatment Principle	Soften hardness and expel *phlegm*; quicken the *blood* and dispel stasis; disinhibit *water* and clear the eyes
Formula 34 plus Formula 38	Er Chen Tang + Xue Fu Zhu Yu Tang Plus and Minus---Citrus & Pinelia Combination + Persica & Cartharmus Combination[9]
	Chen Pi, Fu Ling; Sheng Di Huang, Hong Hua, Chi Shao, Chai Hu, Jie Geng, Chuan Xiong, Niu Xi; Che Qian Zi, Kun Bu

Qi Deficiency from Aging

Symptoms: This advanced stage of ARMD is a result of the long term progression of the dry form. Symptoms result in a gradual decrease of the central vision to the point of legal blindness. The patient is weak overall, has a pale tongue, thin fur or coating, and a weak and slow pulse.

Herbal Treatment

Treatment Principle	Move *qi* and tonify the *blood*
Herb selection is based on the patient's individual needs. Choose 4-6 each time.	Huang Qi, Dang Shen, Dang Gui, Huang Jing, Fu Ling, Bai Zhu, Bai Shao, He Shou Wu, Tu Si Zi, Gou Qi Zi, Nu Zhen Zi, Gan Cao, etc.

Acupuncture Treatment

Ocular Needle: Use ocuzones Upper Warmer (Zone 5) + other zones based on the changes found through observation. If no other diagnostic patterns are observed, use Upper Warmer (Zone 5), Middle Warmer (Zone 8), and Lower Warmer (Zone 13).

Body Points: Baihui (GV 20), Yangbai (GB 14), Sibai (ST 2), Qiuhou (M-HN-8), Taiyang (M-HN-9), Shanzhong (CO 17), Qihai (CO 6), Hegu (LI 4), Taiyuan (LU 9), Xuehai (SP 10), Sanyinjiao (SP 6), Taixi (KI 3), Zusanli (ST 36), Guangming (GB 37), Linqi (GB 41), Xingjing (LR 2), etc. Choose four to six points and alternate use for each treatment.

Seven Star Needle: Dazhui (GV 14) and Huatuo Jiaji. An alternative to these points is to use the following group:

Mingmen (GV 4), Feishu (BL 13), Xinshu (BL 15), Geshu (BL 17), Ganshu (BL 18), Pishu (BL 20), Shenshu (BL23).

Ear Needle: Eye, Lung, Heart, Liver, Spleen, Kidney, Adrenal, etc. Select three to four points and alternate them for each treatment. It is good to leave pellets or seeds on these points which the patients can remove after a few days or if irritation arises.

Scalp Needle: #18 below the occipital line.

New Extra Point Xinming: Dr. Li Pin Qing also obtained good results using strong tonification or rubbing needle technique on the new Extra Point Xinming[10]. (See page 51 for more Information on the use of this point.)

Moxibustion: Alternate between the following four groups:
1. Baihui (GV 20), and Qihai (CO 6)
2. Dazhui (GV 14), Zhongwan (CO 12)
3. Mingmen (GV 4), Quanyuan (CO 4)
4. Zusanli (ST 36), Sanyinjiao (SP 6)

Another moxibustion technique is done using special walnut shell moxibustion glasses.

1. Adding enough water to cover the herbs, boil Ju Hua 30 gm (Chrysanthemum), Gou Qi Zi 60 gm (Lycium fruit) for 30 minutes.
2. Immerse half walnut shells in the boiled solution for at least 24 hours.
3. Fix the soaked walnut shells into specially made eyeglass frames and insert 3 cm long moxa sticks into the moxa holders in front of the frame.
4. After the moxa sticks had been kindled the patient puts on the spectacle frames, and lets his/her eyes receive healing effect from the smoke of the moxa through the heated shells soaked with herbs. The walnut shells must cover the eye orbit. Note that the distance between the burning moxa stick and the walnut shells can be adjusted if the patient feels it is too hot.
5. The patient should close his/her eyelids while doing moxibustion for about 15 minutes, or self-adjust the length of the treatment time. The key point is that the patient is able to tolerate the heat level on his/her eyes.

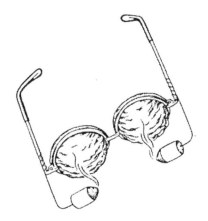

Figure 27 Walnut Shell Moxibustion Glasses

Suggestion: ARMD patients need long term treatment and care and we have to choose the most convenient and beneficial form of treatment for them at different stages of the disease. For example, if the herbal tablets or *wan* form work well, use them instead of the *tang* or tea form. In acupuncture, choose the type of needling treatment that the patient will best accept or else find an alternative needling approach that can obtain the best results.

Common Western and Alternative Treatments for ARMD

Currently in Western medicine, there is no specific treatment for the dry form of ARMD. For the wet form, most ophthalmologists perform treatments such as angiogenesis inhibitors, photodynamic therapy, laser photocoagulation, implantable miniature telescopes, etc.[1] along with the newer Anti-VEGF and ANTI VEGF-A therapy.[11]

Practitioners of alternative medicine have reported they can help the dry form with different kind of treatments such as:

- **Dietary Supplements**: The National Eye Institute's Age-Related Eye Disease Study found that taking a specific high-dose formula of vitamin and mineral supplements significantly reduced the risk of progressing from intermediate to the advanced stage of ARMD. There was no evidence that this formula provided any benefit to patients in the early disease stage. The formula includes Vitamin C 500 mg, Vitamin E 400 IU, Beta-carotene 15 mg, Zinc oxide 80 mg, copper as cupric oxide 2 mg. It is important to note the patient should consult with his/her physician before taking this formula because it may be contraindicated due to other medical conditions or medications.
- **Bone Marrow Stem Cells Transplant** performed by David A. Steenblock, DO.[12]
- **Chelation Therapy** performed by Edward C. Kondrot, MD.[13]
- **Microcurrent Therapy** performed by Gene C. Bruno, L.Ac., OMD.[14]

Prevention

In order to prevent ARMD, people should make an effort to control the risk factors impacting their bodies. However, there are factors such as aging, gender, genes and race that cannot be changed. Their presence should put people on alert to take the best control over those risk factors that can be transformed.

- **Keep the Body in a Balance of *Yin* and *Yang*.** As most people age, it is natural for their bodies to develop a *yin/yang* imbalance, especially due to decreasing liver and kidney *yin*. Liu Wei Di Huang Wan is the best tonic herbal pill to prevent the *yin* from sinking.
- **Self-Massage** around the eyes and on the body points. For technique directions see Chapter 13, pages 145-147.
- **Herbal Patches** around the eyes: Oculax Acupoint Patch for improving eye circulation (Available at www.3t-herb.com).
- **Take MacuCare:** This unique formula combines powerful antioxidants for the promotion of macular health. The contents of one capsule has Taurine 200 mg, Lutein 3 mg, Alpha Lipoic acid 25 mg., and Zeaxanthin 130 mcg. MacuCare is available from PhysioLogics in Colorado, U.S.A. Note that all their products are only sold to licensed practitioners.
- **Ocuvite:** Vitamin and mineral nutrition for the eyes. This formula contains Lutein 5 mg, Zeasanthin 1 mg, Omega-3 fatty acids (EPA 160 mg, DHA 90 mg), Vitamin C 150 mg, Vitamin E 30 IU, Zinc 9 mg, and Copper 1 mg. Ocuvite is from BAUSCH + LOMB, Rochester, NY 14609, USA. Be aware that this company manufactures many different eye care nutrition formulas with similar ingredients - the main difference is in the dosage.

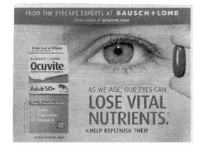

Figure 28   Ocuvite Eye Nutrition

Chinese Herbal Diets

Tonify Liver and Kidney: Especially good for the senior with a sore back and weakness in the knees.

Treatment Principle	Tonify liver and kidney
Diet 1	Gou Qi Zi and Shan Yu Rou Congee
	Gou Qi Zi 9 gram, Shan Yu Rou 9 gram plus glutinous rice 100 gram.

Tonify Spleen and Boost *Qi*. This soup is especially good for the senior who feels fatigue and has loose bowels.

Treatment Principle	Tonify spleen and boost *qi*
Diet 2	Ren Shen Chicken Soup
	Ren Shen 15 gram, Huang Qi 30 gram with a small chicken to make soup
Depending on the person's condition use	Dang Shen or American Ginseng in place of Ren Shen

Tonify Spleen and Kidney. This pudding is good for dizziness and tinnitus, frequency of bowel movements in the early morning and nocturia.

Treatment Principle	Tonify spleen and kidney
Diet 3	Shan Yao + Gou Qi Zi Pudding
	Shao Yao 150 gram, Gou Qi Zi 15 gram with Honey 30 gram.

Suppress Liver *Yang* and Clear Vision. This tea is especially good for lowering elevated triglyceride levels and high blood pressure.

Treatment Principle	Suppress liver *yang* and clear vision
Diet 4	Jue Ming Zi Tea
	Stir fry Jue Ming Zi 15 gram to make 3 cups of tea for a whole day
Notes	<ul><li>If patient has constipation and a bitter taste in his/her mouth, do not stir fry.</li><li>If patient only drinks the tea once a day, use 5 gram of Jue Ming Zi.</li><li>Stop if the patient gets loose bowels.</li></ul>

***Qi* and *Blood* Dual Deficiency.** This tea is good for aging accompanied by general weakness.

Treatment Principle	*Qi* and *blood* dual deficiency
Diet 5	Shen Qi Da Zao Congee
	American Ginseng 5 gram, Zhi Huang Qi 15 gram, Da Zao 5 pieces with rice 100 gram to cook for congee
Depending on the person's condition use	Dang Shen or Ren Shen in place of American Ginseng

- In order to have clear vision and live a healthy life, each individual needs to choose his/her correct diet from this list and to eat it often for the purpose of maintaining a balance of *yin* and *yang* in the body and protecting the eyes. These diets are not only good for ARMD, but also aid aging eyes and bodies in general.
- Maintain a healthy weight; exercise daily.
- Do not smoke.
- Limit caffeine intake to a moderate amount.

- Prevent overexposure to sunlight by wearing wide-brimmed hats and high quality sunglasses that offer 99-100% ultraviolet protection.
- Do self-care massage daily. (See Chapter 13, page 145-147 for details.)
- Live a less stressful, forgiving and happy life.
- Follow professional treatments to take care of other medical conditions.
- Visit an ophthalmologist or optometrist for a comprehensive eye exam once a year in order to screen for eye disease.
- Individuals with high risk factors should do a self-check using the Amsler Grid Test often or even daily. Grid and instructions follow:

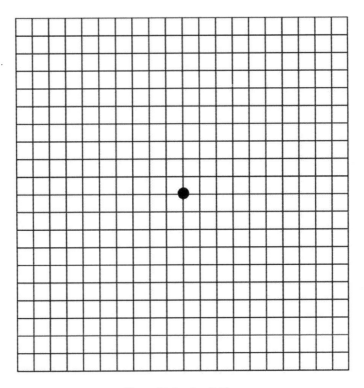

Figure 29 Amsler Grid

Instructions for Using the Amsler Grid

1. Wear the glasses or contact lenses that you normally use for reading.
2. Hold the test grid 13-16 inches away from your eyes.

3. Test each eye one at a time. Cover your left eye and look at the dot in the center of the picture with your right eye. Continue looking at the black dot in the center of the picture and notice whether there are any waves, distortions, or blind spots in the lines.
4. Cover the right eye and repeat the test looking with the left eye.
5. The lines should appear straight and continuous with each eye.

Important: If you notice any waves, distortions, or blind spots in the lines with either eye, please call your optometrist or ophthalmologist as soon as possible.

References

[1] "About Macular Degeneration" by American Health Assistance Foundation, http://ahaf.org/macular, 2/16/2012

[2] "New Strategies for Preventing Vision Loss", *The Johns Hopkins Medical Letter---Health After 50*, Volume 15, Issue 12, February 2004, p. 4-5; "AMD Study: A Feast for the Eyes", Ibid., December 2007, p. 1-2

[3] "A Comprehensive Guide to Macular Degeneration" by Novartis Ophthalmic

[4] 年令相關性黃斑變性的中醫認識, 李學晶等, 中國中醫眼科雜誌, 2008年8月, 第18卷, 第4期, p. 240-241

[5] 現代老年性黃斑變性基礎與臨床研究, (*Current Basic and Clinical Study of Age-Related Macular Degeneration*), 陳松主編, 天津科學技術出版社, p. 630-631

[6] Formula 35: 四物五子丸加減, Ibid., p. 630

[7] Formula 36: 知柏地黃湯加減, Ibid.

[8] Formula 37: 三仁湯, 中醫方劑手冊, p. 235

[9] Formula 38: 血府逐瘀湯, Ibid., p. 192

[10] "針灸新明穴治療老年性黃斑變性 174 例臨床觀察, 聶曉麗等, 針灸臨床雜誌, 1995年, 第11卷, 第1期, p. 22

[11] Brochure, Pacific Cataract and Laser Institute

[12] "Amazing Improvement in Macular Degeneration with Bone Marrow Stem Cells" by David A. Steenblock, DO, Inc., Regenerative News, Spring 2007

[13] "Chelation Therapy and Macular Degeneration", by Edward C. Kondrot, M. D.

[14] "Treatment of Macular Degeneration", by Gene Bruno, OMD, Lac. Presented on WAOMA 2007 Fall membership meeting and seminar, Seattle

CHAPTER NINE

Retinopathy of Hypertension, Arteriosclerosis & Post-Stroke Dysopsia

Gao Xue Ya (Hypertension)
Dong Mai Ying Hua (Arteriosclerosis)
Shi Wang Mo Bing Bian (Retinal Diseases)
Yan Zhong Feng (Eye Stroke)

The development of the diseases of hypertension, arteriosclerosis, and post-stroke dysopsia, is based on primary hypertension. When the arterial pressure of the whole body consistently rises above normal, it causes damage to the walls of the retinal artery, the plasma exudes out of the vessels and infiltrates into the retinal tissue. This can cause the retina to hemorrhage and swell, resulting in the development of some cotton-like white exudates. Depending on the severity of the condition, patients may experience varying degrees of vision loss. The more severe the condition, the worse the eye health is affected.

Factors Relating to these Diseases[1, 2]

Since about 90% of these three diseases develop from primary hypertension, the key must be to prevent hypertension in the first place. It is important to understand and pay attention to these relative factors:

- **Heredity:** Primary hypertension has a significant relationship to genetic makeup. Researchers found that if both parents have hypertension, the

morbidity for their children to develop this disease may be up to 46-50%. If only one parent has it, the morbidity for the children is about 33%.
- Diet
  - Sodium: People with a high intake of sodium and protein have a greater chance of developing elevated blood pressure. Made up of 40% sodium and 60% chloride, salt is an important mineral essential to life that is found in the body and is also used by man for preserving food and stimulating taste buds. However, researchers have discovered that most Americans consume between 6,000 – 12,000 mg of salt daily, an excessive amount that can cause hypertension and other health problems. Recent studies show that for most people, a healthy daily intake of salt is from 500 to 1,000 mg.
  - Potassium: Scientific studies suggest a diet high in potassium can help protect against high blood pressure. It works by stimulating certain hormones and chemicals to release sodium from the blood cells. Some natural foods like bananas contain high potassium levels. Keeping potassium and sodium in the ratio of 3:1 (or even higher for potassium) will benefit the vessels and keep the blood pressure stable.
  - High Protein: Extra protein in the body often leads to weight gain since it can be converted by the liver and stored in the body tissues as fat. Also a diet with too much fat, especially saturated fats, can lead to high LDL cholesterol that blocks the arteries.
- Smoking: Cigarette smoking is dangerous to the health as well as being addictive. Cigarette smoke contains nicotine and carbon monoxide so when the nicotine is inhaled, adrenalin is secreted causing the blood pressure to rise. Also the carbon monoxide, which hemoglobin absorbs over 200 times more readily than oxygen, takes up available binding sites and therefore prevents needed oxygen from passing through the arteries to the rest of the body.[3] This especially causes damage to the heart and brain. Smoking also increases the blood lipid levels which can cause platelets to clot, either resulting in arteriosclerosis or allowing embolisms to develop.
- Alcohol Use: Alcoholic beverages have the impact of elevating blood pressure in general but especially affecting the systolic pressure. Many

researchers believe that alcohol raises blood pressure by directly causing a constriction of blood vessels, which then requires more pressure from the heart to push the blood through the arteries. Another theory is that alcohol stimulates the sympathetic nervous system, resulting in higher pressure. Still other researchers found that alcohol triggers the adrenal glands to release adrenocorticoid hormones causing high blood pressure. The patient in most danger is a heavy alcoholic drinker who ends up with liver and kidney damage causing severe disease. Although some studies show that people who have one or two drinks daily may not cause health damage, people who already have other risk factors should not use alcohol at all. Clinical reports do show a definite rise in blood pressure in people with an alcohol addiction or who have more than three drinks daily.

- **Mental Tension:** People who work or live in a tense environment are more likely to have high blood pressure.
- **Nervous Personality:** People with a nervous personality easily tense up when anxious and if this condition appears often enough, it can raise the blood pressure.
- **Emotional Affect:** A sudden emotion like anger makes blood pressure rise in a person, but other emotions such as panic, terror, fear, or even excessive joy can have the same effect. A person can also cause a rise in blood pressure by holding on to hatred, grief, anxiety or loss for a long period of time.
- **Noisy Environment:** If people work or live in a noisy place for a long time, their sense of hearing weakens which can cause blood pressure to rise.
- **Overweight:** There is a close relationship between being overweight and high blood pressure. About 1/3 of overweight patients have high blood pressure, especially if they have abdominal fat. A simple test for obesity is to stand straight and bend your head down to look at your feet; if the big toe is visible, the abdomen is not yet too serious a health factor in hypertension.
- **Physical Activity:** Exercise may help to lower blood pressure. If a person sits at work daily and lacks other kinds of physical activity, he/she is more likely to have high blood pressure. For seniors, the best exercise is

walking. To keep blood pressure stable, it is recommended to walk at least 30 minutes a day, four times a week.
- **Cold Weather:** If a person living in a cold climate or staying in a cold room does not keep warm enough, he/she can have higher blood pressure than someone living in a warmer climate.
- **Coffee Drinker:** Health experts hold different opinions about coffee and blood pressure. They all agree that after drinking two cups of coffee, a person's blood pressure rises immediately. Some experts say this effect is only temporary while other experts say cutting out caffeine is a sure way to bring blood pressure down. What is agreed upon by all the experts is that everyone has a different tolerance level to caffeine. However, there are some rules from the experts that you should follow in order to avoid triggering high blood pressure and other potential health problems:
    o Do not drink more than two cups coffee daily.
    o Do not drink coffee before going to exercise.
    o People with a heart condition, especially those with arrhythmia, should avoid all coffee.
    o Do not drink coffee before going into a stressful situation such as taking an exam, running in a race, attending a meeting where you will be making important decisions, or being the chief speaker or host of an event, etc.

Factors Relating to Secondary Hypertension

- **Medication:** Blood pressure can also elevate and damage the retina if a patient has taken certain medications for a long period of time or has some previous illness. Some of the common medications such as antihistamines, decongestants, antidepressants, non-steroidal antiinflammatories, corticosteroids, etc. may elevate the blood pressure. Check the package insert of the medicine for the list of possible side effects.
- **Previous Illness:** Diabetes, chronic kidney disease, gout, hyperthyroidism, post-menopausal syndrome, etc. are common diseases of seniors, all sharing one common symptom: high blood pressure. Therefore it is

important to diagnosis whether a patient's high blood pressure is caused by a previously existing illness or if it is a primary problem.

TCM Differential Diagnosis and Treatment[2]

The onset of hypertensive retinopathy may not show any symptoms in the eye, but the patient can already have symptoms of hypertension occurring in his/her body and changes to the retina may be found during the ophthalmoscopy exam by the doctor. After time, the patient gradually loses vision to a noticeable degree. The occurrence of this symptom may eventually become "*wind, phlegm, fire,* and stasis four aspects".

Ascendant Liver *Yang* Transforming into *Wind*

Symptoms: Blurred vision, headache with dizziness, tinnitus, emotional upset, sleeplessness, anger, red face, red tongue, bitter taste, yellow tongue coat, and a string-like and rapid pulse.

Herbal Treatment

Treatment Principle	Calm the liver and suppress excess *yang*
Formula 39	Tian Ma Gou Teng Yin---Gastrodia & Uncaria Combination[4]
	Tian Ma, Gou Teng, Shi Jue Ming (Abalone Shell), Zhi Zi, Huang Qin, Chuan Niu Xi, Du Zhong, Yi Mu Cao, Sang Ji Sheng, Ye Jiao Teng, Fu Shen
For anger and to clear liver *fire* add	Long Dan Cao, Huang Lian
For white exudate on the retina, clear liver *fire*, disinhibit water add	#Chong Wei Zi, Zhu Ling, Xia Ku Cao
For recent hemorrhage and to clear *heat* and cool the *blood*, disinhibit and transform *water* add	Bai Mao Gen

Phlegm and *Dampness* Obstruct the Network Vessels

Symptoms: Blurred vision, heavy-headedness, dizziness, oppressive feeling in the chest, nausea, overweight, pale tongue, greasy coat, string-like and slippery pulse.

Herbal Treatment

Treatment Principle	Harmonize the stomach and expel *phlegm*
Formula 40	Ban Xia Bai Zhu Tian Ma Tang---Pinellia & Gastrodia Combination[5]
	#Ban Xia, Bai Zhu, Tian Ma, Fu Ling, Ju Hong, Cang Zhu, Gan Cao
For headache - to dispel *wind* and release pain add	Man Jing Zi, Fang Feng
For exudates on the retina to quicken the *blood* and dissipate *phlegm* add	Bai Mao Gen, Xia Ku Gao, Yu Jin

Liver-Kidney Deficiency and *Fire* Flaming Upward

Symptoms: Blurred vision with dizziness, tinnitus, irritating *heat* in the *five hearts*, dryness in the mouth and throat, red tongue with a thin and dry yellow coat, string-like fine and rapid pulse.

Herbal Treatment

Treatment Principle	Enrich *yin* and bring down the *fire*; dispel stasis and clear the network vessels
Formula 36 plus 41	Zhi Bai Di Huang Wan + Er Zhi Wan---Anemarrhena, Phellodendron Bark & Cook Rehmannia Formula + Ligustrum & Eclipta Combination
To supplement the liver and kidney *yin*, cool the *blood* and stop bleeding add	Er Zhi Wan[6]
	Nu Zhen Zi and Han Lian Cao

Static *Blood* Obstruction

Symptoms: Vision loss from the disease goes on for a long period. The patient feels a heavy cumbersome headache, damp purple tongue appears with static spots, string-like and tight or rough pulse.

Herbal Treatment

Treatment Principle	Move *qi*, quicken *blood* and clear network vessels
Formula 38	Xue Fu Zhu Yu Tang---Persica & Carthamus Combination
	Tao Ren, Hong Hua, Dang Gui, Sheng Di Huang, Chuan Xiong, Chi Shao, Niu Xi, Jie Geng, Chai Hu, Zhi Ke, Gan Cao
For swelling on the retina, add	Ze Xie, Che Qian Zi, Fu Ling

Long Term Treatment Alternative: Take tablets, pills or patches (Choose Formula 42 or one of the following)

Treatment Principle	Calm the liver *wind*, clear the *heat*, quicken the *blood*, tonify and benefit liver and kidney
Formula 42	Tian Ma Gou Teng Pian---Gastrodia and Uncaria Tablet[7]
	Tian Ma, Gou Teng, Chuan Niu Xi, Yi Mu Cao, Wu Jia Pi, Shi Jue Ming (Abalone Shell), Zhi Zi, Huang Qin, Huai Niu Xi, Du Zhong, Fu Ling, Ye Jiao Teng, Fu shen

- Formula 8: Qi Ju Di Huang Wan.
- Formula 38: Xue Fu Zhu Yu Pian.
- Jiang Ya Jing Tie (Lower Blood Pressure Neck Patch)[8]. This patch contains San Qi, Chuan Xiong, Xi Xin (Asarum), #Wu Zhu Yu (Evodia). Put the patch on Dazhui (GV 14) point and change it daily. The theory is to dissipate external blockages, let the external and internal *qi* move the *blood* and bring down the blood pressure, clearing the vision and the brain in order to prevent the occurrence of stroke.

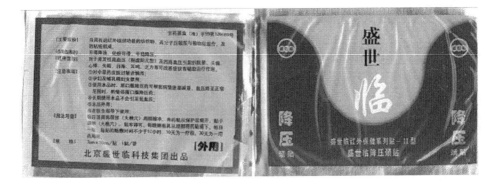

Figure 30 Lower Blood Pressure Neck Patch

Ophthalmoscopic Changes Observed in Hypertension and Arteriosclerosis[9]

In Western science pictures taken of the fundus using fluorescein angiography show very clear changes of hypertensive retinopathy. This is one of the most dramatic signs in ophthalmology. Fluorescein angiography is also an important key for diagnosis since it provides a clear view of the state of the arterioles, particularly reflecting the condition of the vessels of corresponding size in the cerebral circulation.

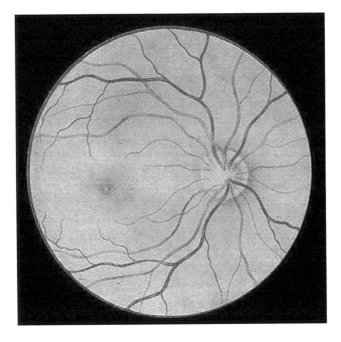

Figure 31 Normal Fundus of Right Eye Seen in Ophthalmoscopic Exam

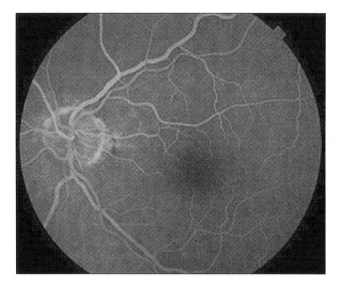

Figure 32 Example of Fluorescein Angiography of an Abnormal Left Eye Fundus

There are many methods attempting to classify the arterial and retinal changes from hypertension and arteriosclerosis but, actually, the changes from these diseases cannot be clearly differentiated. The changes from hypertension gradually move into arteriosclerosis and then the symptoms may overlap and appear at the same time on the retina.

The classification method of Keith-Wagener-Barker that divides these diseases into four groups is one of the simplest but clearest to understand:

1. Retinal arteries are slightly contracted and no longer have a normal shape and size. Patient's blood pressure is slightly higher than 140/90 mmHg.
2. Retinal arteries are narrower at some local locations and some signs show at the intersections where the arteries press on the veins. The patient's blood pressure may be higher than in the first group, yet he/she does not show obvious symptoms. The function of the heart and kidneys is usually normal.
3. Hypertensive retinopathy signs occur: the retinal arteries show significant narrowing like copper wire, the peripheral section of the vein becomes engorged with hemorrhage and cotton-like white exudate appears on the retina. The patient's blood pressure is persistently high and there is

symptomatic evidence of damage from arteriosclerosis found in his/her heart and kidney functions.

4. Changes of retinopathy are worse and the arteries become even narrower like silver wire. The optic disc is swollen and Elschnig maculae spots are present, indicating that the pigmentary epithelial cells have changed due to occlusion blocking the blood supply in the capillary lobules in the choroid layer. Also, there may be more hemorrhages seen on the retina. The patient shows symptoms of severe damage to the brain, heart and kidneys.

Complications of Hypertension

If the patient does not receive treatment on time, complications such as vitreous blood stasis, detached retina and occlusion in the veins of the retina may occur.

Hypertensive Neuroretinopathy[1]

This form of high blood pressure occurs when the pressure rises very high for a short period of time causing severe damage to the vessels in the retina. The main changes seen through the ophthalmoscope are swelling on the optic disc and retina. Other changes that can occur include hemorrhage, cotton-like spots, hard exudates and Elschnig spots.

Symptoms: The patient's vision decreases rapidly accompanied by headache, nausea, vomiting and, in severe cases, convulsion and loss of consciousness. This disease may be caused by the progression of primary hypertension, kidney or endocrine diseases, or high blood pressure syndrome during pregnancy. These cases usually occur before the age of forty.

Treatment: This patient primarily needs to have Western medical treatment. If he/she is also receiving Chinese medical treatment, the protocol used is the same as for primary hypertension.

Remarks: It is important to point out that when the retina still shows fresh hemorrhage or if the retina has detached, acupuncture needling is not applicable. After these symptoms have stabilized, select two to three eye points and four to six body points based on symptom identification such as used for the treatment of other eye diseases. Remember the rule: *"Different diseases may use the same treatment; same diseases may need different ways to treat"*.

When using herbal treatment, it is also very important to be sure the bleeding in the eye has stopped because formulas for the treatment of stanching bleeding are different from those for moving congealed blood. In order to have a clear diagnosis, acupuncturists need to work closely with a patient's ophthalmologist since the doctor can get a clear picture of the retinal vessels using fluorescein angiography and see what is happening inside the eye. The acupuncturist should also listen to the patient's complaints and examine his/her vision carefully before starting any type of treatment.

Post – Stroke Dysopsia

Yan Zhong Feng (Eye Stroke)

Post–stroke dysopsia, a disease of the cerebral blood vessels, is a major complication seen in diseases of the occipital lobe and other parts of the cerebrum. In the clinical setting, it is more common to see patients with stroke occurring in the lateral geniculate body causing post-stroke dysopsia. The occipital lobe, which lies in the back of the skull at the rear of the cerebral cortex, is the visual center of the brain. This lobe is dedicated entirely to the perception and interpretation of visual data delivered from the eye via the optic nerve.

Causes

According to analysis of clinical observation and CT scans, the main cause of post-stroke dysopsia is infarction of blood vessels in the brain. Occasionally it can also be caused by hemorrhage.

Symptoms[10]

A stroke on the right side of any part of the cerebrum causes hemianopia, where the blindness is in the left field of vision of both eyes rather than a complete blindness in only the left eye. The clinical manifestations of post-stroke dysopsia are homonymous hemianopia and a decrease or major loss of visual acuity. A stroke in the occipital lobe can also result in loss of the ability to recognize and interpret visual stimuli such as faces, words, etc. The most common problem seen in clinical cases of dysopsia is infarction at the lateral geniculate body area, although bleeding can be another cause. The patient may present with left limb paralysis and can also lose part of his/her field of vision as shown in Figure 33.

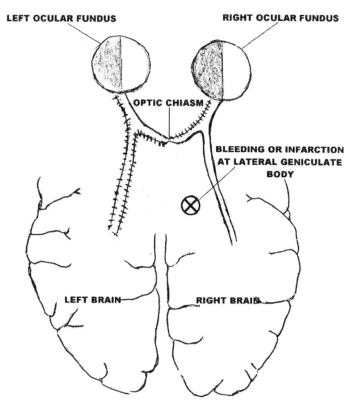

Figure 33 Left-Sided Homonymous Hemianopia Scotoma

In cases of severe stroke where there are body symptoms in addition to the dysopsia, both the patient and doctors may not immediately pay attention to the eye condition due to the urgent need to first address and stabilize the more serious body symptoms. Most patients only start to complain about the dysopsia later after they have been stabilized and then finally become aware of the difference in their vision.

In some cases, a patient experiences transient ischemic attack (TIA) on the eye, suffering a sudden blurring, dimming or even full loss of vision. In addition to the eye symptoms, most episodes of TIA have other symptoms such as weakness, numbness or paralysis, slurred or garbled speech, dizziness and loss of coordination. All episodes usually subside within 5 to 20 minutes and rarely continue for more than a few hours. Because TIAs do not result in permanent neurological deficits, people tend to ignore them. However, people who have repetitive episodes of TIA can eventually develop a stroke. An acupuncturist should know that a TIA symptom showing on the eye is an important warning sign of stroke, and must urge his/her patient to immediately seek medical attention.

Stroke Only Attacking the Eye

There are some rare cases where stroke only attacks the eye. Symptoms include the loss of parts of the visual field depending on where the blockage is located and the type of neurological damage that has occurred.

TCM Differential Diagnosis and Treatment[11]

As with the conditions described above, most patients with post-stroke dysopsia do not seek out acupuncture during the best time to receive treatments. One report in the Shanghai Journal of Acupuncture and Moxibustion, April 2003, Volume 22, No. 4, described treatment of post-stroke eye symptoms. Dr. Zhang Yulian, *et.al.* from the Acupuncture Department of Second Hospital Affiliated with Tianjing College of Traditional Chinese Medicine, China, reported that treatment of 36 cases obtained satisfactory results that were proven by rheoencephalogram and intraorbital rheogram.

Treat post-stroke dysopsia as sequelae symptoms.

Herbal Treatment

Treatment Principle	Tonify *qi* and quicken *blood*, dispel stasis and clear the *luo*
Formula 43 Use this formula first for early stage	Bu Yang Huan Wu Tang---Astragalus and Chinese Peony Combination[12]
	Huang Qi, Dang Gui Wei, Chi Shao, *Di Long, Chuan Xiong, Tao Ren, Hong Hua

Treatment Principle	Dispel stasis and clear vessels, transform turbidity and dissolve fat
Formula 44	Jiang Dan Gu Chun Pian---Crataegi Citrus Fruit Tablet[13]
	Sheng Shan Zha, Gou Qi Zi, Ju Hua, Kun Bu, Shou Wu, Yi Mu Cao, Hong Hua, Huang Jing, Ze Xie, Dang Gui, Chuan Xiong, Ling Zhi

Acupuncture Treatment

Scalp Needle: Insert one needle at the center of the occipital tuberosity and insert two other needles one centimeter bilaterally to this center point.

Filiform Needle: Yangbai (GB 14) →Yuyao (M-HN-6); Taiyang (M-HN-9), Sibai (ST 2), Jingming (BL 1). Treatment is given once per day, one course consisting of five treatments. A total of four courses is administered with a two-day break between each successive course.

Add in GV 20 and distal points depending on the differential diagnosis.

Seven Star Needle: Begin by tapping very lightly around the eye orbit, then increase the tapping intensity and time as the patient tolerates more. *Do not* tap hard enough to cause bleeding!

Prevention of Hypertension, Arteriosclerosis and Stroke

The key to preventing arteriosclerosis and post-stroke dysopsia is to simply take preventive action against hypertension. We have to accept that we cannot change some hypertensive factors such as age, gender, family history, race and prior health history. People in any of these high risk groups should take early action against those factors that can be changed in order to prevent getting hypertension.

General Rules for Stroke Prevention

- Consume a healthy diet that includes low fat foods, low protein, and is high in vegetables and fruits. Pay attention to limiting your salt intake to not more than 2,000 mg per day.
- No smoking, no alcoholic beverages and no caffeine (or a very limited intake).
- Keep up an exercise routine and stay at a healthy weight.
- Relieve stress and tension, keep your emotional state peaceful and stable.
- Try to live in a comfortable environment and avoid a long stay in a cold place.
- Treat ongoing diseases and watch for any medication that has a side effect of causing high blood pressure. Diabetes patients should pay special

attention to keep their blood pressure lower than 120/70 mm Hg. while healthy people should stay within the range of 135-140/85-90 mm Hg.

Prevention Methods

- Balance your *yin* and *yang*, and prevent deficiency of liver-kidney *yin*.
    - Formula 26: Liu Wei Di Huang Wan (Tonify liver and kidney *yin*).
    - Formula 45:

Treatment Principle	Emphasis on tonify kidney *yin*
Formula 45	Zuo Gui Yin---Restore Left Kidney Decoction[14]
	Shou Di Huang, Shan Zhu Yu, Shan Yao, Fu Ling, Gou Qi Zi, Zhi Gan Cao

- For borderline blood pressure use one of the following:
    - Formula 8: Qi Ju Di Huang Wan.
    - Du Zhong Pian (Eucommia Tablet).
    - Jiang Ya Jing Tie Patches (Lower Blood Pressure Neck Patch). Refer to page 101.
- If cholesterol level is borderline, use one of the following:
    - Jiang Dan Gu Chun Pian or Wan, Formula 44, manufactured by Guang Ci Tang. Used for high blood pressure and high triglycerides.
    - Eat oatmeal in the morning.
- If only the triglycerides are borderline or slightly high, use one of the following:
    - Herbal Tea: Shan Zha 9 mg, Ju Hua 9 mg, Jue Ming Zi 6 mg. Make enough tea to drink throughout the day or use it at least three times daily. If a patient has loose bowels reduce the dose; if diarrhea occurs you can omit the Jue Ming Zi from the formula. If the tea upsets the patient's stomach, dilute it or reduce the amount of Shan Zha used.
    - Hawthorn Berries 565 mg capsule. This is Shan Zha powder, manufactured by Puritan's Pride, U.S.A. (www.Puritan.com).
    - Omega-3 Fish Oil 1200 mg soft gel.

Transient Ischemic Attack (TIA) Alert[15]

An acupuncturist should be familiar with the seven common TIA symptoms that occur suddenly but only linger about 5 to 20 minutes before subsiding without any residual damage to the body. TIAs are an important warning sign of an impending stroke and warrant prompt medical attention. In fact, some people have repetitive episodes of TIAs in the days or weeks before a stroke occurs, and one third of those who experience a TIA have a stroke within five years. Recognition and treatment of the causes of a TIA may help to prevent a stroke and its complications.

The Seven Common TIA Symptoms

1. Dimness or loss of vision, particularly in one eye.
2. Sudden weakness, numbness, or paralysis of the face, arm or leg.
3. Loss of speech, trouble talking or understanding speech.
4. Unexplained dizziness, unsteadiness, or sudden falls.
5. Sudden severe headache.
6. Disorientation, confusion, or memory loss.
7. Balance or coordination problems that may fluctuate over a few days.

Dr Zhang Wencai suggested using the following herbal formula for the effective treatment of TIAs.[16]

Herbal Treatment

Treatment Principle	Harmonize the stomach and expel *phlegm*
Formula 40	Ban Xia Bai Zhu Tian Ma Tang---Pinellia & Gastrodia Combination

A practitioner may add more herbs depending on individual symptoms. For convenience to patients, both *pian* and *wan* forms are available.

Self-Care Before the Occurrence of Stroke

TIA Self-Test

Note: Patients with shoulder problems or pain in the shoulder, elbow and wrist should be excluded from doing this test as results will be inaccurate.

1. With closed eyes, extend both arms straight out with palms turned upward, holding them in that position as long as possible. See which arm drops down first. The side that drops first indicates weakness and a greater risk of a future stroke occurring on that side.
2. With closed eyes, extend the right arm with just the index finger straight. Then move your arm so this finger touches the tip of the nose, increasing the speed of the movement in increments to see at what point the finger misses its target. Next repeat the exercise with the left index finger. If the finger misses touching the tip of the nose on one side sooner than on the other, it indicates that there is a greater risk of future stroke on that 'weaker' side.
3. With closed eyes, straighten both arms in front of your body. With index fingers straight and pointing at each other, touch the tips together. Then increase the speed of the movement in increments to see if one side drops and misses touching the other finger tip. The finger that drops indicates there may be a risk of stroke on that side in the future.

Other Self-Care Methods

- Self-massage. Refer to Chapter 13, pages 153-157 for directions.
- Use herbal string or pen moxibustion. Light up the end of the herbal string and quickly touch the point, imediately removing without burning the skin. Repeat three times. Note that there is a possibility of a light burn, but the scar will disappear after a few days. Use this technique on San Yin Jiao (SP 6) and Xuangzhong (GB 39). The moxibustion pen uses herbal paper covering the treatment points. Touch the paper with the moxa pen and immediately remove it without burning the paper or extinguishing the lighted tip of the pen. Repeat

3-5 times. Using this method, neither the paper nor the skin is burned. Following treatment, the moxi Pen is extinguihed by placing it in the glass tube provided. Instructions are included in the moxipen box.

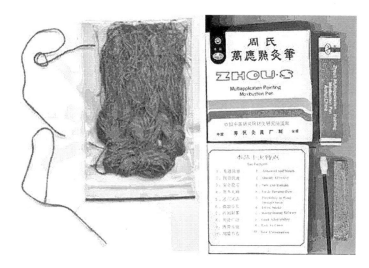

Figure 34 Herbal String (Left) and Pen Moxa (Right)

- Use either a stimulating device, or try the Blood Pressure Depressor machine.

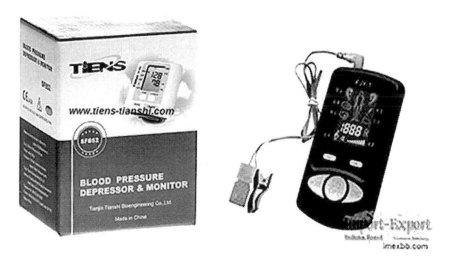

Figure 35 Blood Pressure Depressor and Monitor

- Supplements

- o Stroke experts at the John Hopkins Medical Center suggest taking Vitamin B6 1.7 mg, B12 2.4 mcg and Folic Acid 400 mcg daily. Note that these are approximate dosages.[17]
- o Baby Aspirin 81 mg taken daily, every other day or one to two times a week depending upon the individual.
- Diet: Soup made from Celery Root and Da Zao (Red Date) each 15 pieces; eat daily.

Suggested reading: *Acupuncture for Stroke Rehabilitation* by Hoy Ping Yee Chan, *et.al.*, Chapter 8 on prevention. This section was written by Miranda Taylor, L.Ac.

References

[1] "How High Blood Pressure Can Affect Vision", *Johns Hopkins Medical Center, White Paper for Vision*, 2004, p. 35

[2] 中醫學 (下冊), 河北醫學院主編, 人民衛生出版社, p. 104-107

[3] http://orthosmoke.org/index.php/doc/Carbon%20Monoxide

[4] Formula 39: 天麻鉤藤飲, 中醫方劑手冊, 江西中醫學院附屬醫編, 江西人民出版社, p. 93

[5] Formula 40: 半夏白術天麻湯, Ibid., p. 214

[6] Formula 41: 二至丸, Ibid., p. 151

[7] Formula 42: 天麻鉤藤片, 中醫成方臨床指南, 廣慈堂特效超濃縮丸總覽, 修訂本三, 康業公司, p. 129, K105

[8] Jiang Ya Jing Tie, 降壓頸貼: ForeStar International, U.S.A

[9] 眼底病影像診斷圖譜, 王光璐主編, 北京科學技術出版社, p. 220-222

[10] Gerard J. Tortora, *et.al. Principles of Anatomy and Physiology*, 5th Edition, Harper & Row Publishers, New York, p. 384-386

[11] 頭針加眼周穴治療中風后視覺障礙36例, 張玉蓮等, 上海針灸雜志, 2003年4月, 第22卷, 第4期, p. 6-7

[12] Formula 43: 補陽還五湯, 中醫眼科學, 廣卅中醫學院主編, 上海科學技術出版社, p. 126, #110

[13] Formula 44: 降膽固醇片, 中醫成方臨床指南, 廣慈堂特效超濃縮丸總覽, 修訂本三, 康業公司, p. 145, K119

[14] Formula 45: 左歸飲, 中醫方劑手冊, 江西中醫學界院附屬醫院編, 江西人民出版社, p.147

[15] "Treating a Hidden of Cause of Stroke", *The John Hopkins Medical Letter*, 1996 March, p. 3

[16] 半夏白術天麻湯加味治療中風先兆106例報道, 張文才, 甘肅中醫, 2001年, 第14卷, 第6期, p. 28-29

[17] "Stroke Protection Via Vitamins", *Johns Hopkins Medical Center, White Paper for Hypertension and Stroke*, 2005, p. 41

CHAPTER TEN

Retinopathy of Diabetes

Diabetic Retinopathy (DR),
Xiao Ke Mu Bing (Eye Diseases from the Thirsting and Wasting Disease)
Yun Mu Yi Jing (Cloud and Fog Move into the Eye)
Shi Zhan Hun Miao (Blurred Vision as Mist)
Bao Mang (Sudden Blindness)

Diabetic retinopathy is a group of eye diseases resulting from chronic high blood glucose syndrome that eventually causes changes to the patient's retina. These changes include the development of microaneurysms, occlusion in small arteries, the growth of newly formed vessels changing to fibrous tissue, and retinal detachment. If left untreated, these overall changes can result in vision loss leading to blindness. According to research reports, nearly half of all patients with diabetes develop some degree of this condition during their lifetime. The longer a person has diabetes the greater the risk, so this is a very common eye disease seen in seniors.[1]

In recent years, due to unhealthy dietary habits, the morbidity of diabetes has increased, which causes a similar increase in the morbidity of diabetic retinopathy. For both health practitioners and senior patients, this is an important issue to take note of and to take action on for the prevention of blindness.

Western Medical Symptoms and Diagnosis [2,3]

Diabetic retinopathy is classified as two forms, the non-proliferative form (NPDR) and the proliferative form (PDR).

Non-Proliferative Form (NPDR)

In most patients, the NPDR form which occurs in both eyes either does not affect vision at all or the patient may experience only slightly blurred vision in the early stage. In some cases even after dilating the pupil and doing an ophthalmoscopic exam, the practitioner cannot clearly detect any changes to the retina, nor do they find any small dot hemorrhages, microaneurysms, or the hard exudates that usually appear first on the posterior pole. A better method for diagnosing NPDR is to use a fundus fluorescein angiogram (FFA) to detect changes on the posterior pole where microaneurysms can be found and marked leakage of dye from them are seen. As the disease progresses, vision slowly gets worse. Treatment is most effective when given at this early stage. When the retina begins swelling enough to involve the macula, loss of central vision occurs. In the advanced stage the retina begins to show a mixture of exudates, ischemia and edematous macula. Retinal vein changes are the primary sign used to determine the severity of diabetes.

If occlusions of the capillaries and small arteries develop enough to create ischemic areas, there is no effective treatment that can be given to regain vision. This non-proliferative form may continue to progress into the proliferative form.

Proliferative Form (PDR)

In the early stages of the PDR form, the patient may be symptomless. Abnormal new vessels may form anywhere in the fundus but the main tendency is to form from the disc and around the posterior pole.

This early asymptomatic period of PDR is a problem because the patient loses valuable time to receive treatment. As the disease progresses, hemorrhages may appear on the surface of the retina and even in the vitreous humor, and there also may be many newly formed abnormal vessels growing inside the vitreous chamber. After any blood has been absorbed, these vessels change to white fibers on the retina or in the vitreous humor and lead to scarring, causing retinal detachment and potentially resulting in permanent vision loss.

TCM Differential Diagnosis and Treatment[3]

If the disease of *Xiao Ke* (diabetes mellitus) has continued for a long period without symptomatic treatment and the blood glucose remains at a high level, it may cause *Xiao Ke Mu Bing* (diabetic retinopathy). Both NPDR and PDR forms result from chronic illness that causes deficiency and influences the condition of the vessels, resulting in stasis and bleeding due to *blood heat*.

The pathogenesis of this situation is *qi* and *yin* dual deficiency. *Qi* deficiency can first lead to *blood* stasis, then the vessels lack nourishment leading to blurred vision. The root is *qi* and *yin* deficiency while the branch is *qi* stagnation and *blood* stasis. As these conditions reciprocally affect each other, *phlegm* and *dampness* develop or *yin* and *blood* deficiency result in bleeding on the retina and into the vitreous humor, resulting in severe vision loss.

Yin Deficiency and *Dry-Heat*

Symptoms: The patient experiences blurred vision, thirst and drinks plenty, feels hunger and eats frequently, experiences weakness in the lower back and knees, mouth is dry, tongue is red with little coating and the pulse is deep and fine.

Fundus Exam: microaneurysms and hemorrhagic spots and exudates can be seen.

Herbal Treatment

Treatment Principle	To enrich *yin* and moisten the dryness, cool the *blood* and transform the stasis
Formula 36	Zhi Bai Di Huang Tang Plus and Minus---Anemarrhena and Phellodendron Combination
To cool the *blood* and transform stasis add	Chi Shao
To moisten and enrich fluid add	Mai Men Dong, Shi Hu, Xuan Shen
For fresh bleeding add	Ce Bai Ye, Da Ji, Xiao Ji, etc.

Dual Deficiency of *Qi* and *Yin*

Symptoms: The patient may see floaters in front of his/her eyes, experience blurred vision, fatigue and shortness of breath, be too tired to talk, have an expressionless face, a dim complexion, dry throat, spontaneous perspiration, and a burning sensation of the *five centers*; have a pale swollen tongue, and an empty and weak pulse.

Fundus Exam: Retinal swelling, edematous macula, hemorrhagic spots and exudates can be seen.

Herbal Treatment

Treatment Principle	Enrich *qi* and nourish *yin*
Formula 26 + Formula 6	Liu Wei Di Huang Wan + Sheng Mai San
For Retinal hemorrhages add	San Qi powder, Qian Cao
For spontaneous perspiration add	Huang Qi, Fu Xiao Mai

Dual Deficiency of Spleen and Kidney

Symptoms: The patient sees floaters in front of the eyes and has blurred vision; his/her body is either thin or is thin but edematous, complexion is yellowish or blackish; experiences dizziness with tinnitus, tiredness in the low back and knees, impotence and polyuria at night. In the advanced stage the patient has a decreased amount of urine, a pale face, swollen and pale tongue with a white coating, and a deep and weak pulse.

Fundus Exam: Retinal swelling and edematous macula, hemorrhagic spots and exudates.

Herbal Treatment

Treatment Principle	Warm *yang* and boost *qi*, enrich kidney
Formula 18	Jin Gui Shen Qi Wan (also called Fu Gui Ba Wei Wan)--- Eight Flavor Rehmannia Pills (or use the same herbs to make Shen Qi Tang)

Static Blood Occlusion in Eye

Symptoms: The patient has poor vision, sees black shadows moving in front of the eye or even experiences partial vision; dizziness or vertigo, chest oppression, numbness in the limbs; dusky purple tongue with static spots; has a string-like and rough pulse.

Fundus Exam: New growth retinal vessels and proliferative inner layer membrane have developed and hemorrhages are connected together as large pieces can be seen.

Herbal Treatment

Treatment Principle	Quicken the *blood* and transform stasis; clear the vessels and brighten the eye
Formula 38	Xue Fu Zhu Yu Tang Plus and Minus
For fresh bleeding add	San Qi powder, Da Ji, Xiao Ji, Ce Bai Ye, Qian Cao, Xian He Cao, etc.
For static blood spots and pieces add	Dan Shen, Yu Jin, Ji Xue Teng

Phlegm–Stasis Occlusion in Vessels

Symptoms: The patient may see black shadows moving in front of the eyes with accompanying vision loss, be overweight or exhibit heaviness in his/her body, have a dusky purple color on the lips and the tips of the limbs; tongue is dusky purple with static spots and has a thick and greasy coating; pulse is string-like and slippery.

Fundus Exam: Retinal swelling with exudates, newly formed vessels and hemorrhages, proliferative membrane on the retina and vitreous body developing together; detached retina can be seen.

Herbal Treatment

Treatment Principle	Dry the dampness and expel *phlegm*; quicken *blood* and dispel stasis
Formula 31	Wen Dan Tang Plus and Minus
To transform *phlegm* and resolve depression add	Dan Shen, Yu Jin, #Dan Nan Xing, Hong Hua, Tao Ren, etc.
To quicken *blood* and transform the proliferative membrane	Hai Zao, Kun Bu

Dr. Chen Yu, *et al.*, suggested using another method to identify the key for treatment by focusing on these three appearances: deficiency, *heat* and stasis. He created a Standard Formula for different kinds of deficiency.[4]

Herbal Treatment

Treatment Principle	Tonification
Formula 46 For *yin* and *blood* deficiency	Standard Formula
	Huang Jing, Shan Yao, Sha Shen, Mai Dong, Sheng Di Huang, Gou Qi Zi
For *qi* deficiency add	Huang Qi, Bai Zhu
For *yang* deficiency add	Ba Ji Tian, Xian Ling Pi
For fresh bleeding add	Pu Huang *E Jiao, Yi Mu Cao
For exudates add	Dan Shen, Chi Shao, Huai Niu Xi, Yu Jin
For hard exudates on the macula add	Shan Zha, *Ji Nei Jin
For retinal swelling add	Fu Ling, Yi Yi Ren
For blood stasis, bleeding more than three months, newly formed vessels, proliferative member and scar development add	Dan Shen, Huai Niu Xi, *Chuan Shan Jia, *Di Long, Kun Bu, Hai Zao

Note: The above information is taken from the article "TCM for Treatment of Diabetic Retinopathy Based on Syndrome Differentiation", published in the *Journal of Traditional Chinese Ophthalmology*, April 2009, Volume 19, Number 2.

Modifying Formulas Using Mi Meng Hua

None of the formulas for the herbal treatment of diabetic retinopathy included the herb Mi Meng Hua. This herb is usually used for an infection of the outer eye. However, there are many articles where the authors state that Mi Meng Hua is helpful for diabetic retinopathy as well. So if the above herbal formulas do not work as well as expected, you may try adding Mi Meng Hua to the formula to see if it helps.

Acupuncture Treatment

Treatments should be given before hemorrhage appears or after any bleeding has been stablized.

Ocular Needle: Choose any ocuzones with observable changes. If none, use the standard triple warmer zones: Upper Warmer (Zone 5), Middle Warmer (Zone 8), Lower Warmer (Zone 13) or choose other group zones such as Kidney (Zone 3), Liver (Zone 6) or Spleen (Zone 11).

Scalp Needle: #18 under the occipital line, #1 frontal midline.

Filiform Needle: Jingming (BL 1), or Qiuhou (M-HN-8), Shenting (GV 24), Taiyang (M-HN-9) for adjustment to move the *qi* and *blood* around the eye area. Do not apply stimulation after insertion.

Also add in one of the following points:
Quchi (LI 11), Yinlingquan (SP 9) or Xuehai (SP10), Taixi (KI 3), Taichong (LI 3);

or choose: Hegu (LI4), Zusanli (ST36), Sanyinjiao (SP 6).

Diet[5]

Diabetes patients have varying degrees of *yin* deficiency so for both prevention and long-term self-care, attention to diet is very important to use in conjunction with other treatments. Taking the herb Shan Yao is the first dietary choice to make. In this chapter Shan Yao was used in three important herbal formulas - Zhi Bai Di Huang Tang, Liu Wei Di Huang Wan and Dr. Wu Danyi's Standard Tonification Formula (written in the article by Dr. Chen Yu, *et. al.*). Shan Yao can also be used in a diabetic's diet for effect. However the diabetic patient should be careful and also control his/her intake of carbohydrates and fatty foods.

1. Shan Yao 100 gm. Steam to cook it well and eat before a meal; it is best to eat it often.
2. Shan Yao and Tian Hua Fen each 15 gm to make tea; drink often. This tea is good for relieving thirst.
3. Pumpkin 250 gm to make soup, take once or twice daily.
4. Pumpkin 500 gm - cut into pieces, fry and eat often.

5. Spinach root 250 gm, Ji Nei Jin (chicken's stomach) and rice 100 gm to make congee; eat many times a week.
6. Spinach root 90 gm, and dry Ji Nei Jin 15 gm to make soup. Use twice daily.
7. Bitter melon tea bag or dried pieces to make tea; drink often.
8. Gou Qi Zi 10 gm to make tea; drink often throughout the day.
9. Drink Tang Zhi Di Tea daily. This is a powder in a tea bag made from wild guava fruit and leaves.
10. Pig pancreas one piece, corn hairs 30 gm, Zhi Shi (Fructus Aurantii Immaturus) 15 gm + 5 bowls of water, cook down to a volume of one bowl; eat often.

Prevention

The most important part of prevention is to control diabetes as much as possible to minimize the risk of developing retinopathy.

1. **Healthy Diet and Exercise:** This is the key for controlling the blood sugar level in the body. Seniors should pay attention to keep the *yin* and *yang* balanced in their bodies and to especially prevent the *yin* from sinking. Take Liu Wei Di Huang Wan, and alternate with the diet information above.
2. **Special Teas:** For prevention or for people with borderline glucose levels, drink bitter melon tea or Tang Zhi Di Tea (wild guava fruits and leaves) daily.
3. **Self-check Your Fasting Glucose:** A healthy senior should have this test done every three to six months; for the senior whose fasting glucose is borderline, check monthly; for the early stage diabetic patient, check weekly; for a patient who has gone beyond the early stage, check daily.
4. **Check A1C Hemoglobin in the Lab:** The A1C checks a person's average hemoglobin level over a three month period. For a healthy senior, check once a year; for the senior whose fasting glucose is borderline, check twice yearly; for diabetic patients, check quarterly.

5. **Control Blood Pressure:** The best blood pressure for the diabetic patient is 120/70 mmHg.
6. **Control Serum Lipid Levels:** The majority of diabetic retinopathy patients have hypertension and hyperlipemia, so having the blood pressure and lipid levels well under control indirectly helps to prevent diabetic retinopathy.
7. **Do Not Smoke:** Smoking has a close relationship with both hypertension and hyperlipemia so smokers have more chance to develop diabetic retinopathy.
8. **Herbal Patch**: You can try the herbal foot patch distributed by ForeStar International, Inc. U.S.A. The purpose of this patch is to help the pancreas restore normal, healthy function. The patches are placed on the soles of the feet overnight. Note that this is typically a long-term treatment so recheck your blood sugar after about a month to determine how effective this method is in your case. The six main herbs used in the foot pads are Sheng Ma, Ge Gen, Chai Hu, Hong Hua, Dang Gui, and Wu Zhu Yu.

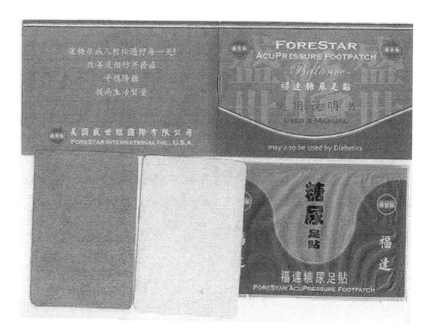

Figure 36 ForeStar Diabetes Footpatch

9. **Fundus Exam:** Once a year a patient should have a fundus exam done with dilated pupils. The earlier diabetic retinopathy is detected, the less the risk for vision loss.
10. **Massage or Tapping:** Do frequent massage, tapping or needling on Yishu (M-BW-12), Pishu (BL 20), Shenshu (BL 23), Zusanli (ST 36), and Taixi (KI 3) to move *qi* and enrich *yin*. Yishu has also proven effective in controlling the function of pancreas.

References

[1] "Diabetic Retinopathy", *Johns Hopkins Medical Center White Paper for Vision*, 2004, p. 41-46

[2] Diabetic Retinopathy brochures, American Academy of Ophthalmology

[3] 中老年眼病中西醫結合治療學, 楊光主編, 華中科技大學出版社, 中國, 武漢, p. 232-236

[4] 中醫藥治療糖尿病視網膜病變辨証論治概述, 陳郁等, 中國中醫眼科雜誌, 2009年, 4月, 第19卷, 第2期, p. 122-123

[5] 漫話糖尿病與食療, 錢桂華, 藥膳食療研究, 2000年, 第4期, p. 7

CHAPTER ELEVEN

Occlusion

Bao Mang (Sudden Blindness)

Chinese Medicine categorizes occlusion of either the central retinal artery or vein as belonging to the list of *Bao Mang*, a symptom that can result from many internal eye or body conditions. In Western medicine this is considered an emergency eye disease. It occurs more in people in late middle age and seniors, especially those with hypertension, cervical arterial sclerosis, coronary heart disease or diabetes. The accepted thought is if the patient does not receive proper treatment of an arterial occlusion within one hour of onset, the prognosis is poor. For this reason it is important for practitioners to recognize the onset and early stages of this disease.

Central Retinal Artery Occlusion (CRAO)

Bao Mang (Sudden Blindness)

Occlusion of the retinal artery can be caused by obstruction or blockage of the retinal vascular lumen by an embolus, thrombus, or by inflammatory or traumatic vessel wall damage or spasm. During a blockage, oxygen does not flow to the retina and may result in severe loss of vision.[1]

Causes of Arterial Occlusion According to Western Medicine[2, 3, 4]

1. **Changes to the Inner Layer of the Arterial Wall:** Retinal arteries and veins become smaller. Thrombosis forms at the different parts of the central retinal artery due to endarteritis, sclerosis, degeneration, narrowing, etc.
2. **Thromboembolism:** Embolisms can result from issues in distant parts of the body such as arterial plaques in the cervical artery or heart valves, cholesterol, fibrin, calcium, cancer, fat, medication, air, etc.
3. **Other Possible Causes:** These include vasospasm, viscosity of the blood stream due to abnormal conditions of the blood cells, high IOP, high orbital pressure, etc.

TCM Pathogenesis of CRAO[3]

The occurrence of sudden blindness can arise from four kinds of pathogenesis.

1. **Damage from Emotional Effects:** The patient has a violent temper and gets extremely angry, or damage results from emotional stress caused by overwhelming sadness and grief.
2. **Food and Drink Intake:** The patient consumes too many fatty, spicy foods or drinks too much wine and, as a result, may develop *phlegm* and *heat* rising upward to the eye.
3. **Physical Weakness from Aging:** Deficiency of liver-kidney *yin* causes *yang* hyperactivity, the abnormal raising of *qi* and *blood* blocks the blood flow causing stagnation in the arteries.
4. **Deficiency of Heart *Qi*:** This condition decreases heart strength for moving the blood properly. This in turn causes the blood stream to flow more slowly finally resulting in *blood* stasis forming in the arteries.

TCM Differential Diagnosis and Treatment[3,4]

Symptoms: Sudden blindness in one eye without experiencing pain and visual acuity reduces to CF (counting fingers) or HM (hand motion). The patient may experience temporary amaurosis (sudden blindness) before this disease onset. The pupil dilates and LR (light reaction) delays or even vanishes. If the patient receives both Chinese and Western treatments in time, there is a good chance that he/she will regain at least some degree of vision.

Qi and *Blood* Stagnation

Symptoms: The patient has emotional depression with liver *qi* stasis, sudden loss of vision, dizziness and headache, purple tongue, and a string-like and rough pulse.

Herbal Treatment

Treatment Principle	Quicken the *blood* flow and clear the orifices
Formula 47	Tong Qiao Huo Xue Tang---Clear Orifices and Quicken *Blood* Formula[5]
	Chi Shao, Tao Ren, Hong Hua, Chuan Xiong, Lao Cong (old green onion), Sheng Jiang, Hong (Da) Zao

Phlegm Heat Rises Upward

Symptoms: Patient loses vision suddenly, feels heaviness and vertigo in his/her head, has chest pressure, nausea and no appetite, sticky phlegm with bitter taste, tongue coating is yellow and greasy, pulse is string-like and slippery.

Herbal Treatment

Treatment Principle	Expel *phlegm* and clear the vessels; quicken *blood* and open orifices
Formula 48	Di Tan Tang---Rinse *Phlegm* Formula[6]
	#Ban Xia, #Dan Nan Xing, Ju Hong, Zhi Shi, Fu Ling, Ren Shen, (Shi) Chang Pu, Zhu Ru, Gan Cao, Sheng Jiang, Da Zao

Liver *Wind* Internal Stirring Upward

Symptoms: Patient loses vision suddenly, experiences dizziness and tinnitus, tidal redness in face, dysphoria and anger, sleeplessness with dreams, bitter taste with red tongue and yellow coat, and a string-like pulse.

Herbal Treatment

Treatment Principle	Calm liver and extinguish the *wind*; clear vessels and open the orifices
Formula 39 For hyperactivity of *yang*	Tian Ma Gou Teng Yin
Formula 49 For liver *wind* internal stirring	Da Ding Feng Zhu Plus and Minus---Settle Down the *Wind* Formula[7]
	Gan Di Huang, Bai Shao, Mai Dong, Wu Wei Zi, Gan Cao, (Huo) Ma Ren, *E Jiao, *Ji Zi Huang, *Sheng Gui Ban, *Sheng Mu Li, *Sheng Bie Jia

Qi Deficiency and *Blood* Stasis

Symptoms: Eye symptoms are the same as with the other patterns, patient has weakness of *qi* and does not like to talk, fatigue, pale face, pale tongue with purple spots, rough and moderately weak pulse that pauses at regular intervals.

Herbal Treatment

Treatment Principle	Boost *qi* and quicken *blood*; clear vessels and brighten the eye
Formula 43 to treat the branch until stable and the second part of **Formula 11** to treat the root	Bu Yang Huan Wu Tang; Si Wu Tang

Blood Stasis

Symptoms: This type may be caused by hypertension. The patient has poor vision, dizziness, heart palpitations, fatigue and weakness, poor or no appetite, may have either loose bowels and diarrhea or abdominal distention and constipation, sore and tight limbs, possible edema in the lower legs, pale tongue with purple spots, and a rough and deep pulse.

Herbal Treatment

Treatment Principle	Quicken *blood*, dispel stasis and clear the *luo mai*
Formula 43	Bu Yang Huan Wu Tang Plus and Minus

Acupuncture Treatment

Scalp Needle: #18 under the occipital line.

Ocular Needle: First use ocuzones with observed changes. If none are seen, choose standard Kidney (Zone 3), Upper Warmer (Zone 5), Liver (Zone 6). You may need to add on Heart (Zone 9).

Filiform Needle: Around eye points Qiuhou (M-HN-8)[8], Jingming (BL 1). Body points are selected based on the differential diagnosis.

Ear Needle: Points for Eye, Vision (Mu) 1 or 2 and also select more points based on the differential diagnosis.

Seven Star Needle: Lightly tap 3-5 times around the outside of the orbit, increasing up to around 30 times if the patient can tolerate it. Add in the five back shu points + Geshu (BL 17).

Dr. Chen Wei Li, *et al.,* from the Ophthalmology Hospital of the Chinese Medicine Research Academy, China, suggested that for better results give a combined therapy of the five methods listed below to treat the early stage of CRAO.[8]

1. Acupressure on The Eyeball: With the eyelid closed apply pressure with alternating index fingers to the upper eyelid of the affected eyeball 60 times.

2. **Oxygen Therapy:** Inhale a low flowing amount of oxygen for 1 hr/day, for one week.
3. **Point Injection:** Ling Guang Zhen (Complex Anisodin Injection) 1 cc. Use for point injection on Taiyang daily, 10 days as one course.[8]
4. **Herbal Treatment:**

Treatment Principle	Quicken the *blood* and transform stagnancy
Formula 33	Tao Hong Si Wu Tang + *Shui Zhi, *Quan Xie
For edema on retina add	Che Qian Zi, Ze Xie
For high blood pressure add	Tian Ma, Gou Teng
For constipation add	Da Huang

5. **Prescription drugs:** Used for quickening the *blood*, dilating the arteries and dispelling the stagnation.

Prevention

If a patient comes to an acupuncturist with sudden blindness, it is important to immediately refer that patient to an ophthalmologist, as emergency medical treatment is needed to save his/her vision. The accepted thought is that prognosis is poor if the patient does not receive the proper treatment within one hour. In the meantime, applying acupressure to the affected eyeball may have the valuable benefit of moving the blockage farther down to the smaller arteries, thus minimizing damage to the retina.

Following emergency treatment, you may apply acupuncture.

For pathogenesis and prevention guidelines see hypertensive retinopathy on pages 104-105.

Ophthalmoscopy Changes Seen in CRAO[3, 9, 10]

The optic disc is a pale color, swollen with an unclear edge. The retinal arteries become smaller, making it harder to find the small branches (because they are all terminal branches). The corresponding area of the retina which receives the blood supply from the affected artery is swollen and its color changes to a creamy white. It appears shaped like a tongue or rectangle. A positive sign for CRAO is when the color of the macula shows as a cherry-red spot and the central light reflection has vanished.

If the patient does not receive appropriate treatment, the optic nerve will atrophy, then the optic disc will change to a pale color with a clear edge. If the affected area is the connective branch of the ciliary retinal artery, a tongue-shaped pink area appears at the side of the disc extending to the macular area. In this case, the patient may recover some degree of vision.

Complications

1. Retinal hemorrhages.
2. Central retinal vein occlusion.
3. Occurrence of secondary glaucoma.

Other Medical Exams To Help Clarify a Diagnosis of Occlusion[3]

- Vision Field: The field of vision is damaged, constricted or even changed to tunnel vision depending on the degree and location of the occlusion.
- FFA: Fundus fluorescein angiography shows the actual condition of the vessels.
- ERG: Electroretinography shows a falling b wave.

Central Retinal Vein Occlusion (CRVO)

Bao Mang (Sudden Blindness)
Shi Zhan Hun Miao (Blurred Vision as Mist)

This is a very common retinal vascular disease that usually occurs in late middle age and in seniors. It is more common than CRAO and the symptoms typically occur in one eye only, showing as blood stasis, hemorrhage and swelling. The chance of visual recovery with certain forms of CRVO has a poor prognosis.

Causes & Pathological Changes of CRVO According to Western Medicine[11, 12]

1. **Changes to the Vessels:** Due to high blood pressure, arteriosclerosis, diabetes, and infectious diseases from other parts of the body such as periphlebitis, endocarditis, or septicemia.
2. **Changes of the Composition of the Blood:** The quality of protein in plasma, hyperlipidemia, erthrocythemia, and leukemia.
3. **Hemodynamic Changes:** The blood stream in the retina is slow and due to that and the thickness of the blood, there is an increased chance of coagulation.

    Note that in general, any of the three changes noted above cannot be looked at as a single cause for CRVO, since they usually are mixed together in a complicated pattern caused by vein occlusion.

4. **Categories:** The modern method of investigation using FFA had shown that CRVO can be subdivided into two broad categories, either hemorrhagic or stasis. Severe vision loss results from the hemorrhagic type while less severe vision loss results from the venous stasis type. With the stasis form, full recovery of vision can be expected.

TCM Differential Diagnosis and Treatment[12]

Liver-Gallbladder *Fire* Flaming Upward

Symptoms: Vision loss resulting in a sudden downgrade to CF or HM, headache, heart irritation, sleeplessness, loses his/her temper so easily gets angry or depressed, dry mouth and bitter taste, red tongue with yellow coat, and a string-like and rapid pulse.

Fundus Exam: There is a layer of red color from either retinal hemorrhage or the vitreous humor, and the vessels of the retina may not be visible in the ophthalmoscopy exam.

Herbal Treatment

Treatment Principle	Clear and drain the liver *fire*
Formula 50	Long Dan Xie Gan Tang---Gentiana Combination[13]
	Long Dan Cao, Sheng Di Huang, Dang Gui, Chai Hu, Mu Tong, Ze Xie, Che Qian Zi, Zhi Zi, Huang Qin, Sheng Gan Cao

Stagnant *Qi* and *Blood* Stasis

Symptoms: Disorders of *qi* can cause *qi* and *blood* stagnation. The patient has vision loss and feels pressure on the eyes, headache, feels distension pain in the chest and hypochondrium, has loss of appetite and belching, tongue is faded red with purple static spots and a thin white coat, the pulse is string-like or rough. Some patients may have *qi* deficiency with palpitations and a rapid or fine pulse.

Fundus Exam: There is a lot of blood in the retina with engorged, swollen and twisted veins. This is an excess pattern in the branch.

Herbal Treatment

Treatment Principle	Move the *qi* and relieve depression
Formula 51 Use if there is still fresh hemorrhage on the retina	Chai Hu Shu Gan Tang---Bupleurum & Cyperus Combination[14]
	Chai Hu, Xiang Fu, Zhi Gan Cao, Zhi Ke, Bai Shao, Chen Pi

Note that if the bleeding has stopped but the clot still looks pink, add in Formula 33 (below). Formulas 51 and 33 can be used together.

Treatment Principle	Quicken the *blood* and dispel stasis
Formula 33 Use after the retinal hemorrhage stabilizes	Tao Hong Si Wu Tang---Persica, Carthamus + Angelica Four Combination
	Tao Ren, Hong Hua, Dang Gui, Chuan Xiong, Shu Di Huang, Bai Shao

Treatment Principle	Quicken the *blood* and dispel stasis; clear the *luo* (vessels)
Formula 43 When the patient has deficiency of *qi* add	Bu Yang Huan Wu Tang---Astragalus & Red Peony Combination[17]
	Huang Qi, Chi Shao, Dang Gui Wei (tail), Chuan Xiong, Tao Ren, Hong Hua, *Di Long

Yin Deficiency Causes Hyperactive *Fire*

Symptoms: The patient has had vision loss for a period of time, experiences dizziness and tinnitus, lumbago and weak knees, burning sensation in the *five centers*, red cheeks and lips, dry throat and mouth but no desire to drink, red tongue with minimal coating, and a fine and rapid pulse.

Herbal Treatment

Treatment Principle	To enrich *yin* and bring down *fire*; cool and stanch the *blood*
Formula 36	Zhi Bai Di Huang Tang Plus or Minus
Retina still has fresh bleeding add	Bai Mao Gen, Di Yu Tan (ash), San Qi Fen (powder), Han Lian Cao
Retinal hemorrhage has stanched and changed to static spots add	Chuan Xiong, (Chuan) Niu Xi, Dan Shen
Hyperactive liver *yang*, dizziness add	Bai Shao, *Long Gu, *Mu Li, *Gui Ban

Dual Deficiency of Heart and Spleen

Symptoms: The disease is chronic, symptoms come and go, retinal hemorrhage, vision has not recovered, the face is pale and without spirit or expression, fatigue and lack of strength, too lazy to speak, intense throbbing heart palpitations, poor appetite, thin sloppy stool; the tongue is pale, pulse is empty and weak.

Herbal Treatment

Treatment Principle	Support and nourish heart and spleen; boost *qi* and stop chronic hemorrhage
Formula 52	Gui Pi Tang Plus and Minus---Angelica, Ginseng & Longan Combination[15]
	Dang Gui, Ren Shen, Long Yan Rou, Bai Zhu, Fu Shen, Suan Zao Ren, Mu Xiang, Gan Cao, Yuan Zhi
To support *blood* and stanch blood flow add	*E Jiao, San Qi Fen, *Xue Yu Tan

NOTE: If the patient is actively hemorrhaging, do not apply acupuncture. After the bleeding has stopped you can do body needling by selecting points based on the differential diagnosis. Needles around the eye area should be gently and carefully inserted without any form of stimulation.

Ophthalmoscopic Changes Seen in CRVO[17]

With the occlusion occurring in the retinal vein, the side of the vein distal from the occlusion becomes engorged and varicose, looking like a dim purple-colored sausage. Because of the lack of oxygen, infiltration of the vessel wall increases causing exudates, retinal edema and hemorrhages to develop. These changes can cause retinal atrophy or degeneration as well as narrowing of the retinal arteries due to reflex constriction.

CRVO combining with edema in the macula increases the chance of central vision loss. The optic disc changes to a red color with an unclear edge and there are many flame-like hemorrhages spreading out from the side of the optic disc. In a severe case, there are many fragile abnormal newly formed vessels that can easily leak, allowing blood to spread into the vitreous chamber and mix with vitreous humor. You can see this condition by looking through the pupil with the naked eye.

Complications

1. Blood in the vitreous chamber (vitreous hemorrhage).[17]
2. Secondary Glaucoma: Researcher Zhang Wei Rong reported that about 40%-80% CRVO cases can result in secondary glaucoma.[18]

Prevention

Development of CRVO has a close relationship to an imbalance of the *yin* and *yang* of the liver, kidney, spleen and heart. The most important key for preventing this condition is to keep this balance functioning well and to follow the prevention rules for hypertension to stay healthy.

References

CRAO References

[1] http://eyewiki.aao.org/Retinal_Artery_Occlusion

[2] 現代眼科手冊, 人民衛生出版社, 楊鈞主編, p. 255-256

[3] 中老年眼病中西醫結合治療學, 華中科技大學出版社, 楊光主編, p. 219-223

[4] 針藥并施治療視網膜動脈阻塞, 田開愚, 中國中醫急症, 1999年, 第8卷, 第6期, p. 285

[5] Formula 47: 通竅活血湯, 中醫方劑手冊, 江西中醫學院附屬醫院, 江西人民出版社, p. 191

[6] Formula 48: 滌痰湯, 中老年眼病中西醫結合治療學, 華中科技大學出版社, 楊光主編, p. 363

[7] Formula 49: 大定風珠, 中醫方劑手冊, 江西中醫學院附屬醫院, 江西人民出版社, p. 91

[8] 中西醫結合治療中央動脈阻塞療效觀察, 陳偉麗等, 中國中醫眼科雜誌, 2007年, 12月, 第17卷, 第6期, p. 334-335

[9] 眼底病圖譜 (*Atlas of Ocular Fundus Diseases*), 張惠蓉主編, 人民衛生出版社, p. 237-251

[10] 眼底病影像診斷圖譜, 王光璐主編, 北京科學技術出版社, p. 187-195

CRVO References

[11] 現代眼科手冊, 人民衛生出版社, 楊鈞主編, p. 246-249

[12] 中老年眼病中西醫結合治療學, 華中科技大學出版社, 楊光主編, p. 224-229

[13] Formula 50: 龍膽瀉肝湯, Ibid., p. 359

[14] Formula 51: 柴胡舒肝湯, Ibid., p. 363

[15] Formula 52: 歸脾湯, Ibid., p. 359

[16] 補陽還五湯治療氣虛血瘀型高血壓視網膜靜脈阻塞療效觀察, 阿琴等, 中國中醫急症, 第9卷, 第5期, 2000年, 10月, p. 232

[17] 眼底病影像診斷圖譜, 王光璐主編, 北京科學技術出版社, p. 201-202

[18] 眼底病圖譜 (*Atlas of Ocular Fundus Diseases*), 張惠蓉主編, 人民衛生出版社, p. 252-280

CHAPTER TWELVE

Presbyopia
Lao Shi (Old Eye's Vision)

Presbyopia, the difficulty of focusing on close objects such as when reading, is an eye condition caused by aging. It isn't even considered an ametropia or eye disease because during the aging process, the lens gradually becomes thicker and more rigid and is less able to change its shape to bring close objects into focus. The cells of the lens continue to change even though the eye stops growing in the early teen years. In addition, the connective muscle of the ciliary body attached to the lens weakens during the aging process. This muscle helps the lens to adjust its amplitude in order to create a clear image on the retina. The combination of these two factors causes presbyopia.

Symptoms[1,2]

Even though symptoms vary from person to person there are three general age groups for onset of presbyopia symptoms.

- **Emmetropia** (normal vision) - symptoms start occurring at 40 - 45 years of age.
- **Myopia** (nearsightedness) - depends on the strength of glasses worn by the patient and may appear many years later. The stronger the prescription strength, the longer it takes to appear.
- **Hyperopia** (farsightedness) - symptoms appear at a young age.

Some people feel that the symptoms of presbyopia develop suddenly, but actually the condition takes years to progress. A person with blurred vision at the normal reading distance of one foot or 30-33 cm, may be unaware of how far away he/she is holding reading material in order to make it easier and clearer to see. Without taking care of this problem, an aging person may begin to experience other symptoms such as eye fatigue, dizziness, nausea and headache.

Western Medical Treatment[1, 2, 3]

In Western medicine there are no preventive measures for presbyopia and the accepted treatment is to prescribe reading glasses, bifocals, trifocals, progressive lenses or contact lenses by doctors of optometry. However, there currently is some research being done on using surgery to correct the condition.

The effects of presbyopia constantly change the ability of the crystalline eye lenses to focus properly for clear vision. As a result, eyeglasses or contact lenses must be changed periodically in order to maintain good vision and avoid the onset of side effects. If a person frequently changes his/her eye glasses and still does not see as well as expected, other eye diseases such as cataracts should be considered and a comprehensive eye exam is needed.

TCM Differential Diagnosis and Treatment[4]

Symptoms: Chinese medicine considers that the symptoms of presbyopia are not just age-dependent, but are also related to the constitution of the person based on TCM differential diagnosis. If a person matches one of the patterns below, he/she may show symptoms sooner than a healthy person.

Heat attacks Kidney causing Kidney *Yin* Deficiency

Herbal Treatment

Treatment Principle	To first clear *heat*, then tonify kidney *yin*
Formula 53	Di Zhi Wan Plus or Minus[5]
	Tian Men Dong, Sheng Di Huang, Zhi Ke, Ju Hua

Acupuncture Treatment

Ocular Needles: First choose zones based on observed changes. If there are no obvious changes use ocuzones Kidney (Zone 3) or Lower Warmer (Zone 13), Upper Warmer (Zone 5);

Plus add in points: Quchi (LI 11), Taixi (K 3).

Filiform Needles: Chengqi (ST 1), Taiyang (M-HN-9), Hegu (LI 4), Zhaohai (K 6) or alternate with this second group: Jingming (BL 1), Sibai (ST 2), Quchi (LI 11), Taixi (K 3).

Plus add in

Seven Star Needle: Tapping on Dazhui (DU 14), Shenshu (BL 23), Pangguangshu (BL 28).

Dual Deficiency *Yin* of Liver and Kidney

Herbal Treatment

Treatment Principle	Enrich and nourish liver and kidney *yin*
Formula 8	Qi Ju Di Huang Wan Plus or Minus

Acupuncture Treatment

Ocular Needles: Choose zones based on observed changes. If none, select Kidney (Zone 3), Liver (Zone 6); plus choose body points: Taixi (K 3), Xingjian (LV 2) or Taichong (LV 3).

Filiform Needles: Tongziliao (GB 1), Zanzhu (BL 2), Sanyinjiao (Sp 6), Zhaohai (K 6).

or alternate with this second group: Jingming (BL 1), Yangbai (GB 14), Taixi (K 3), Xingjian (LV 2) or Taichong (LV 3);

Plus add in

Seven Star Needle: Tap on Ganshu (BL 18), Shenzhu (BL 23).

Dual Deficiency of *Qi* and *Blood*

Herbal Treatment

Treatment Principle	Tonify *qi* and *blood*, harmonize *yin* and *yang*
Formula 11	Ba Zhen Tang Plus or Minus

Acupuncture Treatment

Ocular Needles: Choose zones based on observed changes. If none seen, use Upper Warmer (Zone 5), Middle Warmer (Zone 8), Lower Warmer (Zone 13);

Plus choose Zusanli (ST 36), Sanyinjiao (SP 6).

Filiform Needles: Jingming (BL 1), Tongziliao (GB 1), Zusanli (ST 36), Sanyinjiao (SP 6);

or alternate with this second group: Chengqi (ST 1), Sizhukong (SJ 23), Hegu (LI 4), Xuehai (SP 10);

Plus add in

Seven Star Needle: Tap on five Back Shu Points plus Geshu (BL 17).

Diet

As we age it is good for eye health to consistently take the herb Gou Qi Zi which improves liver and kidney *yin*. You can clean 10 to 15 pieces and chew them, use them for tea, add to other food dishes or use them to make soup.

Another important nutrition for eye health is lutein, found in green leafy vegetables such as broccoli, green beans, peas, Brussels sprouts, cabbage, kale, spinach, etc. By frequently eating these foods, eye aging problems can be slowed or entirely prevented.[6]

Prevention

Although Western medicine has no way to prevent presbyopia, there is a way that can help delay its onset or even eliminate the need to wear reading glasses in a lifetime.

I (Hoy Ping Yee Chan) learned an eye exercise for the prevention of presbyopia while attending the International Congress of Chinese Medicine & Acupuncture Towards Worldwide Recognition held in Singapore in 1992. This eye exercise, taught by a doctor from the College of TCM, Lanzhou, Gansu, strengthens the three pairs of eye muscles that help shape the eyeball, pulling it longer to adjust the amplitude accommodation. In the case of myopia (being nearsighted), the eyeball is already longer so someone with nearsightedness is more likely to get a less-severe case of presbyopia; also myopia shows up later in life than in those who are farsighted or have normal vision.

Consider that the eyeball is like a poached egg. If outside force is applied, its shape changes, much like what happens to an inflated balloon when it is touched. The three pairs of eye muscles work together by pushing or pulling the eyeball, changing the amplitude accommodation which in turn results in a clear image on the retina. This exercise can make the eyeball lengthen slightly as the muscles get stronger.

I obtained some good results using this exercise both on myself and many of my patients. The level of improvement depended upon what age the exercises were started and how consistently a daily routine was followed. It is important to start doing this exercise around the age of forty or before the symptoms of presbyopia first appear. If the exercises are started after the symptoms have already occurred or if you are already wearing corrective glasses, any effect on presybiopia is minor but would still be helpful for the eyes in general.

Eye Exercise for the Prevention of Presbyopia

I have modified the following directions for this eye exercise for improved results.

1. Keeping your head still and looking straight ahead, hold an extended index finger horizontally about one foot in front of your nose. Then move your arm upward to forehead height while keeping your eyes focused on the finger. Next, following the finger by only moving your eyes, move

the arm downward until level with your nipples,. Begin with 20 -30 repetitions and then add more until you reach about 60. You can also alternate using the other arm and finger to do the same kind of up and down motion. In this way, both shoulders are exercising at the same time. When only one side is used, it can tire too soon. This action strengthens both the superior and inferior rectus muscles of the eyes.

2. Rub your palms together as quickly as you can until they turn hot, then immediately use them to cup both closed eyes. Hold until the palms no longer feel warm. Repeat this action three times. This exercise allows your eyes to rest after step one.

3. Extend your index finger on either hand straight up, holding it about one foot in front of your nose. While keeping the head straight and still, use only your eyes to follow the finger as your arm moves back and forth from left to right at ear level. Repeat this exercise 20 to 30 times, working up to 60 repetitions.

   If this action is too hard for you to do, start at the center of the body in front of your nose and only use the index finger of the left arm, moving it back and forth from your nose to left ear 20 to 30 times.

   Then follow the right index finger from the midline in front of your nose as you move your right arm back and forth between your right ear and the midline for another 20 to 30 times. Work up to 60 repetitions. This action strengthens both the medial and external rectus muscles of the eye.

4. Repeat step two.

5. Straighten the right index finger and hold it about one foot in front of the right eye. Keeping your head straight and stationary, use both eyes to follow the moving finger as if writing a horizontal figure 8 or the infinity symbol. Repeat 20 to 30 times, then repeat the same movement with your left arm working up to 60 repetitions. This action strengthens both the superior oblique and inferior oblique muscles of the eye.

6. Repeat step two.

7. Keeping your head straight and still, focus both eyes through a window at a distant object for one to three seconds. Immediately change your focus

to either your index finger or a pen held about one foot in front of your nose. Continue to change your visual focus from the distant target to the close finger or pen as fast as possible and as many times as you can by dropping the pen or finger from view, then moving it back up into your line of sight. At the start of this exercise, if you feel it is too difficult to change visual focus fast and often, start slower by lengthening the focus time to four to five seconds, and only do 10 to 15 repetitions to avoid dizziness or nausea. After you become used to this action, increase the speed and number of repetitions. For best results do this exercise 100 to 200 times. This exercise forces all three pairs of eye muscles to work together, and strengthens the power of these six muscles to adjust the shape of the eyeball resulting in a clear retinal image.

8. Repeat step two and then give your whole body a good rest.

Note: The instructions say to do this exercise 20-30 times, working up to 60, but for even better results feel free to do it as many times as possible. Just don't overdo the exercise to the point of feeling nausea or dizziness.

References

[1] Brochure of American Optometric Association on Presbyopia

[2] 眼科學, 毛文書主編, 人民衛生出版社, p. 170

[3] 現代眼科手冊, 楊鈞主編, 人民衛生出版社, p. 572-573

[4] 中老年眼病中西醫結合治療學, 楊光主編, 華中科技大學出版社, p. 317-319

[5] Formula 53: 地芝丸, Ibid., p. 360

[6] *PDR for Nutritional supplements*, Sheldon Saul Hendler, PhD. MD, Chief Editor, Published by Medical Economics, Thomson Healthcare, p. 281

CHAPTER THIRTEEN

General Prevention for Aging Eyes

Like other parts of the body, the eyes gradually deteriorate due to aging with the result of weakened vision. Although this is a normal process, if we start taking care of the eyes before age forty, there is a chance to slow down the deterioration. There are some people who don't have any vision problems as they age; they can still thread a sewing needle without any help or need to wear eyeglasses. Therefore it is totally worthwhile to try these harmless Chinese traditional preventive eye care methods for yourself or to share them with your patients.

Preventive Methods for Eye Care

In general, do not overuse your eyes. Avoid reading, viewing your computer, or watching television for longer than one hour at a time. After an hour of these types of activities, be sure to rest and do either method #2 or #3 as described below. These methods help to both protect your eyes and benefit vision.

1. **Relax the Eyes While Looking:** Face a window and look at a distant target (a green object is best) for about one minute. Then close your eyes and relax for about 20 seconds. Now repeat looking and relaxing two more times. The purpose of this exercise is to help the eye muscles to relax even though they are working to give you a clear image on the retina. Do it at least twice daily or even more if you have time.
2. **Warm Up the Eyes:** Rub your palms together as quickly as you can until they turn hot, then immediately place them over your closed eyes and hold until the palms are no longer warm. Repeat these steps twice. This

method warms up the eyes and brings more *qi* and *blood* and nourishment to them. Suggestion: Steps one and two are more beneficial if you do them together.

3. **Remove Blockages:** With eyes closed, use the thumb and index finger to slightly knead the inner part of both eyes at the acupuncture point Jingming (BL 1) for about one minute. Then using either the thumb or index finger, press from the inner corner of the left eye and follow the upper edge of the orbit socket, moving to the outer corner of the eye at the acupuncture point Tongziliao (GB 1). From there press and move the finger along the lower edge of the orbit socket back to the point Jingming (BL 1). If some tender spots are felt, apply slight pressure on those spots for 10 seconds, repeating three times. Usually these tender spots disappear when you do the next round. The purpose of this method is to clear the blockages in the channels and vessels around the eyes, allowing the *qi* and *blood* to move smoothly in order to nourish the eyes.

4. **Strengthen the Eye Muscles:** With eyes closed, circle both eyes clockwise five times, then counterclockwise five times; then close your eyes and let them rest. Doing this method exercises all three pairs of eye muscles, strengthening their amplitude accommodation for adjusting the eyeball.

Here is also another way to achieve this same purpose:

While holding your head and neck steady, look at the Chart #1 in Figure 37 and use both eyes to follow the arrows as they spiral from the outside in to the center. Then look at Chart #2 and follow the arrow from the center of the circle to the outside. Repeat these two movements five times. Note that some people may experience nausea when they do this exercise. If this occurs, close both eyes and rest. In this case, you can also choose to do the exercise described in Chapter 12, pages 145-147.

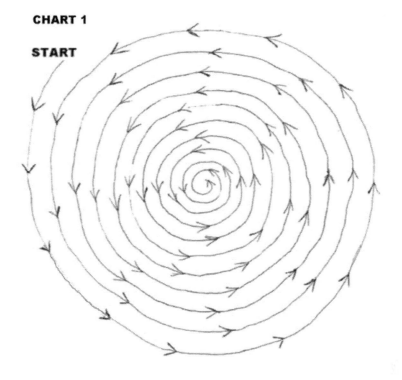

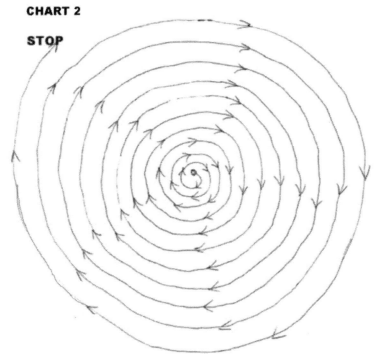

Figure 37 Eye Exercise Chart

5. **Hot Patch on the Eyes:** Wet a small towel with hot water and place it over the closed eyes for about 15 minutes; make it as warm as you can tolerate and keep the temperature stable. Do often, especially if your eyes feel uncomfortable. This method increases the blood flow to the eyes and clears the vessels.

6. **Steam the Eyes:** Choose two or three kinds of Chinese herbs that work to clear *heat*, benefit liver and brighten the eyes such as Ju Hua, Mi Meng Hua, Gu Jing Cao, Xia Ku Cao, Pu Gong Ying, Dan Zhu Ye, Bo He, etc. Put the selected herbs in a pot with enough cool water to cover them and bring it to a boil. After boiling, pour the hot tea into a thermos bottle with an opening of 2.5 -3 inches. Then being careful of the distance your eyes are from the hot steam, close your eyes and let the steam envelop them for five to six minutes. The distance from your eyes to the steam should feel comfortably warm, but not hot or burning. You may reuse the herbs two or three times over the following days by simply warming the tea up again.

7. **Bathe the Eyes:** Dunk your open eyes into a pot of warm water filled with dissolved sea salt.[1] The salt density and the temperature should be at a level you can tolerate for one minute. Raise your head for a few seconds, then immerse your open eyes into the salt water again. Repeat 5 - 6 times, then use fresh, unsalted water to rinse your eyes thoroughly. This method helps to clean the outer parts of the eyes and increases circulation.

8. **Nourish the Eyes:**[2] Eat more dark green vegetables, yellow and orange colored fruits which contain high levels of carotenoids that can defend against some eye conditions. Lutein and zeasanthin, also important for the eyes, are found in spinach, kale, broccoli, green beans, green bell pepper, squash, sweet potatoes, papaya, oranges, mango, peaches, red grapes, etc. A good source for Omega-3 fatty acids is wild salmon, tuna, sardines, walnuts and flaxseed oil. Citrus fruits, tomatoes, strawberries, cantaloupe and yams contain high Vitamin C. Eggs, whole grains, wheat germ, fortified cereals, nuts and nut oils contain Vitamin E. All these foods can benefit eye health. The well-known Chinese herb (also called a fruit) is Gou Qi Zi. Chinese and Western researchers have proven it is the best

nutrition for the eye. The use of it has been mentioned in many chapters in this book so it will not be repeated here.

9. **Correct Lighting and Glasses:** You should avoid reading under too bright a light like sunlight or using a bright computer. Also do not read when it is too dark or dim, or in a moving vehicle. Wear suitable sunglasses to protect your eyes from ultraviolet rays and corrective glasses if needed for good vision.

Note: You do not need to do all these methods at the same time, but it is good to choose a group of three to use for a time and then alternate with another group.

General Preventive Self-Care Method for Senior Health

Traditional Chinese medicine looks at a person as a whole. As such it considers that a person with healthy aging eyes must still have a balance of *yin* and *yang* and *blood* and *qi*, not just isolated in the eyes but throughout his/her entire body. Therefore, doing general preventive health self-care techniques is of the same importance as for eye health prevention methods.

Self-Care Technique

1. With your index, ring and middle fingers follow the pathways of the GV, BL and GB channels, knocking back and forth on the scalp for 91 - 99 times to clear the channels and move the *qi*. Since the head belongs to *yang*, this technique benefits the whole body by raising up the *yang qi*.

2. Using all the fingers on both hands, comb the scalp from the GV channel to the temporal sides of the head for 21 - 31 times to clear the *luo mai* (vessels) and move blood.

3. Use both thumbs to apply acupressure to Fengchi (GB 20) for about 30 seconds; relax the thumbs slightly and rub on the point for another 30 seconds. Repeat these two techniques for a total of 5 - 6 times. This technique benefits the head, nose and eyes.

4. Use both thumbs and massage across the back of the neck from Fengchi (GB 20) passing extra point Anmian (N-HN-54) to Yifeng (TB 17); rub back and forth for two minutes to calm the mind and aid sleep.

5. Use both palms to cover the ears tightly, then quickly release the palms from the ear in order to cause vibration of both ear drums. Do this technique 30 - 40 times. Next, continuing to cover the ears, use your index and middle fingers to knock on the occipital part of the head (called "beating the sky-drum") for 30 - 40 times. This technique also causes vibration on the ear drum. Another method is to firmly place your middle finger on the occipital area of your scalp and then put the index finger on top of the middle finger; next quickly flick the index finger down to the scalp 30 - 40 times. This technique causes a broader vibration affecting the ear drum creating healthy movement and benefitting hearing.

6. Place your middle fingers in front of the ears and index fingers behind the ears and rub up and down for 30 - 40 times or until the skin feels warm. The purpose is to clear the blockages and move the *qi* freely at three points in front of the ear - Ermen (TB 21), Tinggong (SI 19), Tinghui (GB 2) - and two behind the ear - Yifeng (TB 17) and extra point Yilong (N-HN-15). This technique benefits hearing by moving any blockage in all the associated acupuncture points, thus freeing the *qi* of the Triple Warmer, Small Intestine and Gallbladder channels and their linking organs.

7. Use the thumb and index finger to massage both ears going from the inner chamber to the ridge and down to ear lobe until both ears become red and warm. Benefits of this technique include warming up the whole body and moving the *qi* and *blood* freely.

8. Use your index and middle fingers to put pressure at the sides of the spine at Dazhu (BL 11), applying three to four seconds of acupressure and then moving up to Tianzhu (BL 10). This technique should be done in four to five steps, applying three to four seconds of acupressure in each step, then releasing the fingers and moving upward if there are no tender spots. If some points are still tender, do a few more repetitions. The purpose is to

clear blockages in the Bladder channels so the *qi* moves freely in the channels and relieves neck muscle tension.

9. Using your middle, index and ring fingers, move from Shenting (GV 24) and Meichong (BL 3) on both sides down to extra point Yintong (M-HN-3) and Zhazhu (BL 2) bilaterally. Repeat moving up and down about 30 - 40 times or until you feel your forehead turn warm. The purpose is to clear blockages in the Governor vessel and Bladder channel, allowing *qi* to move freely. This technique benefits frontal headache, sinus, and eyes.

10. Use your lower teeth to knock the upper teeth 30 - 40 times, three times daily before or after meals.

11. Use two index fingers to massage both sides of the bridge of the nose for 30 - 40 times; then apply acupressure at Bitong (M-HN-14) and Yingxiang (LI 20), about ten seconds for 5 - 6 times. This technique benefits the nose and sinus.

12. Another massage method is to use the proximal phalangeal joints of the index and middle fingers (bending the fingers creates stronger pressure) and massage the Bladder channel from Fengmen (BL 12) down to Shenshu (BL 23) on the back, moving from upper to lower until your arm gets too tired or you feel that your whole body has warmed up and is comfortable. This massage can be done with the patient clothed but the clothing should not be too thick. This technique benefits general health by clearing the blockages in the Bladder channel and moving the *qi* freely to support increased flow of *qi* and *blood* into internal organs.

13. If someone is constipated, use the palm of the right hand and rub clockwise from the belly button towards the outside 60-100 times. If the patient has diarrhea, do the opposite movement using the left hand and rub counterclockwise from outward towards the belly button 65-99 times.

14. Following the microacupuncture technique ECIWO[3], massage back and forth on the 2nd metacarpal to find any tender point. If one is found, apply acupressure at that point. (ECIWO means Embryo Containing Information Whole Organism.) See the picture below:

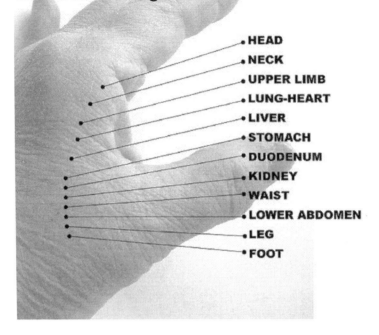

Figure 38 Embryo Containing the Information of the Whole Organism

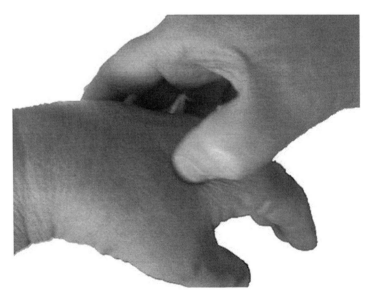

Figure 39 Acupressure Technique for ECIWO Method

15. Use your thumb to follow the pathway of the Pericardium channel on the inside of the upper arm moving from medial down to the distal; then follow the pathway of Triple Warmer from the hand up to the shoulder. Repeat these movements until the skin feels warm to the touch and is slightly pink. The benefit of this technique is to balance *yin* and *yang* of *blood* and move *qi* through the arm channels.
16. Use the thumb to follow the Spleen channel, starting above the ankle and moving up to Yinglingquan (SP 9); then go from Zusanli (ST 36), Yanglingquan (GB 34) and Weizhong (BL 40) moving down to the exterior ankle. Repeat these movements until the skin gets pink and feels warm to the touch. This technique benefits balancing *yin* and *yang* of *blood* and *qi* movement through the leg channels.
17. Apply acupressure to Sanyinjiao (SP 6) for one minute and rub on the point. This technique benefits the three *yin* channels of Spleen, Liver and Kidney and their associated organs.
18. Rub the sole of the foot until it is warm and then apply pressure on Yongquan (KI 1) for 1 minute; rest a moment and repeat two more times. This point is called the second heart of the body and can tonify the kidney and warm up the whole body.

Note: It is best to avoid pressuring the patient to do these self-care methods as he/she should be self-motivated to do them to obtain the benefits.

Because there are many acupressure techniques, a person may not be able to do them all at one time, so they can be spread out over time. Another option is to let the patient select some of the techniques that feel right to him/her.

If the patient is not interested in doing the self-care acupressure, or the practitioner does not have the time to explain them, there is a simple exercise that only takes a minute to demonstrate:

Stand with your arms at your sides and begin gently swinging your arms in sync, back and forth in a continuous motion, slowly increasing the amplitude until they reach shoulder height, about 180 degrees. Repeat at least 100 and up to 500 times or more. This exercise moves the *qi* in the entire body due to the three *yin* and three *yang* hand channels that move through the shoulder region and their association with the three *yin* and *yang* foot channels.

References

[1] 鹽療治百病, 安心編輯部著, 世茂出版社, 2000, 台北, p. 175-188

[2] "Vision" Food to Include in Your Diet, from http://www.brightfocus.org/

[3] 生物全自息診療法, 張穎清, 山東大學全息生物學研究所, 山東大學出版社, 1987

APPENDIX ONE

Introduction to Ocular Diagnosis and Periocular Acupuncture

Source: *Window of Health---Ocular Diagnosis and Periocular Acupuncture*
by Hoy Ping Yee Chan, O.M.D.

Ocular diagnosis and periocular acupuncture is a form of microsystem acupuncture based on traditional Chinese medical theory that the eye connects to the acupuncture channels and the organs of the whole body. In the late 70's, Professor Peng Jingshan of Liaoning College of Traditional Chinese Medicine discovered and developed this unique technique. In 1982, it was evaluated and approved as a new acupuncture therapy by the government of Liaoning Province. Then in 1986, it was recognized by the nation of China. Professor Peng introduced this therapy at the First World Conference on Acupuncture – Moxibustion which was held in Beijing, China in 1987, and then this new therapy spread to the world. In 1996 Hoy Ping Yee Chan, O.M.D. compiled her book *Window of Health---Ocular Diagnosis and Periocular Acupuncture* in order to help share the information she learned both at the conference and time she spent later at Dr. Peng's eye needle research clinic in 1993.

For this book, we have chosen important information required for any acupuncturist to know before applying the technique of periocular needling. That information is found both in this appendix as well as throughout the book.

Finding the Ocuzone Locations

To apply the location of the Eight Octants in clinical practice, ask the patient to lie in a supine position with the head towards north and the feet towards south. Using the face of a clock as an analogy, the first region is at 10:30 -12:00 and is the direction of the Qian Diagram situated on the north northwest of the individual's left eye. Because the left eye belongs to *yang*, the following seven regions are counted clockwise for location. The right eye belongs to *yin* so the order is reversed and counted counterclockwise.

Have the patient look straight ahead. The ocuzones are constructed by first drawing a horizontal line through the two canthi and a vertical line through the center of the pupil. The four resulting sections are bisected equally to form eight regions.

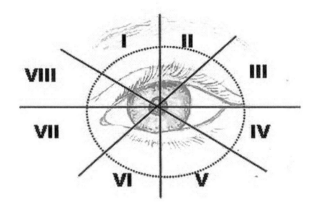

Figure 40 Left Eye Divided into the Eight Regions

Next, divide the five regions I, II, IV, VI, and VII evenly in two. As a result, the original eight regions have now become 13 ocuzones.

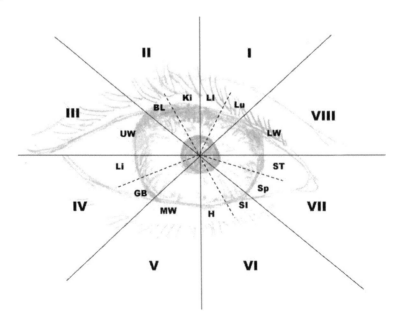

Figure 41 Right Eye Divided into the Eight Regions and 13 Ocuzones

The Eight Regions and Thirteen Zones

REGION	CLOCK	DIRECTION	BAGUA	SYMBOL	FUNCTION	ACU-ZONES	ZANG FU
I	10:30 - 12:00	NNW	QIAN - Heaven	☰	Transmission	1 2	Lung Large Intestine
II	12:00 - 1:30	NNE	KAN - Water	☵	Body Fluid	3 4	Kidney Bladder
III	1:30 - 3:00	ENE	GEN - Mountain	☶	Perineum	5	Upper Warmer
IV	3:00 - 4:30	ESE	ZHEN - Thunder	☳	Purity	6 7	Liver Gallbladder
V	4:30 - 6:00	SSE	XUN - Wind	☴	Nourishing	8	Middle Warmer
VI	6:00 - 7:30	SSW	LI - Fire	☲	Uterine Yang	9 10	Heart Small Intestine
VII	7:30 - 9:00	WSW	KUN - Earth	☷	Foodstuff	11 12	Spleen Stomach
VIII	9:00 - 10:30	WNW	DUI - Marsh	☱	Guanquan	13	Lower Warmer

Figure 42 Table of Eight Regions and Thirteen Zones

The Thirteen Ocuzones

The eight octants make up the thirteen ocuzones on the white part of the eye. Five octants contain one *zang* and one *fu*: I, II, IV, VI, VII. The following shows the organ pairs located in the respective octants.

In the first group, one of each of these pairs is located in half of each of their respective octants.

I—Lung and Large Intestine

II—Kidney and Urinary Bladder

IV—Liver and Gallbladder

VI—Heart and Small Intestine

VII—Spleen and Stomach

Octants occupying whole regions are III, V, and VIII.

III—Upper Warmer

V—Middle Warmer

VIII—Lower Warmer

Important Note: *The 13 ocuzones associated with the eyeball itself are used for diagnostic purposes only, the eyeball is never needled! The extension of the 13 ocuzones into the periocular regions is where actual needling takes place.*

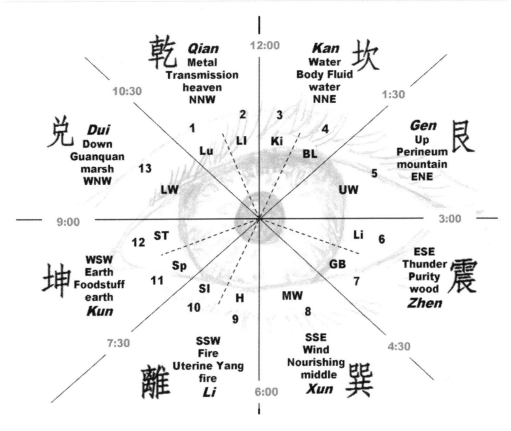

Figure 43 Eight Diagrams, Eight Octants, Eight Regions, Locations, Directions, *Zang-Fu* and 13 Ocuzones On Left Eye

Triple Warmer Theory of Ocular Acupuncture
The Eye and the *Sanjiao* (Triple Warmer, Triple Burner)

The Triple Warmer is a single *fu* governing the movement of *yuan qi*, *water* and *grain*. It frees the waterway. All *essences* and fluids need to pass through this organ to reach the eye and nourish it.

If the function of the Triple Warmer is impaired, the eye does not receive nourishment. If the Triple Warmer waterway is obstructed *dampness* collects, invades the eye and may cause eye diseases.

The Triple Warmer (*Sanjiao*), which vitalizes and coordinates all the body's functions, has three sections: The Upper Warmer, Middle Warmer and Lower Warmer.

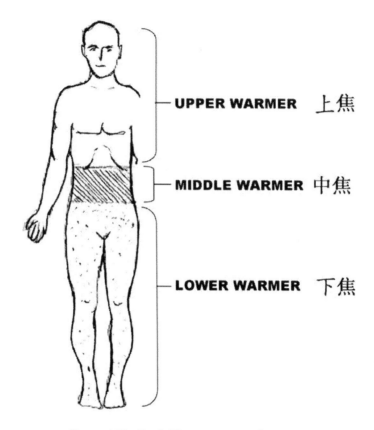

Figure 44 The Triple Warmer Regions of the Body

Miraculous Pivot says, "The Upper Warmer resembles the movement of the fog; Middle Warmer absorbs and transfers; and the Lower Warmer acts as drainage for the excretory system."

In the book *Classical Medical Questions* it is written, "Triple Warmer has a title but no form." Professor Peng points out that in the ocular region, the Triple Warmer should be interpreted in an expanded sense only. The Upper Warmer is located in the area above the diaphragm and contains the chest, upper back, organs, head, neck, and upper extremities. The Middle Warmer is the area located between the diaphragm and umbilicus and contains the upper and middle abdomen and organs. The Lower Warmer is the area located below the umbilicus and includes the lower abdomen and its organs, lumbar region and the lower extremities.

These defining boundaries aid in the discernment of clinical symptoms for ocular diagnosis and periocular needling. The microacupuncture system based on these Triple Warmer boundaries treats all disorders.

1. The Upper Warmer treats problems of the chest, including the heart, lungs, ribs, esophagus, trachea, head, neck, the five sense organs and the upper extremities.
2. The Middle Warmer treats disorders of the middle section of the spine, epigastrium, stomach, spleen, liver, gallbladder, pancreas and small intestine.
3. The Lower Warmer is used for any illness of the lumbar sacral region, pelvic cavity, buttocks, urogenital problems, small intestine, large intestine and disorders of the legs and feet.

The Principle of Therapeutic Selection of Ocuzones

1. By observing the eye for pathological or color changes.
2. According to the location of the disease in the Triple Warmer.
3. Along the channel which corresponds to the occurring symptoms.
4. Based on differentiation of the syndrome.
5. By referencing the exterior-interior relationship.
6. Using the theory of contralateral acupuncture.

Periocular Needling Technique

- **Needle Selection:** The Chinese brand needle gauge for periocular needling technique ranges from #29 to #38 and should be 0.5 *cun* in length. The key is that the bigger the gauge, the better the effect.
- **Patient Position:** The patient is put in supine position for treatment and should be calm and comfortable before needling.
- **Insertion:** The acupuncturist should use the thumb and index finger of one hand to tighten the eyelid on the selected zone and push the eyeball

away from the zone for protection. The other hand holds the needle for insertion. Being precise within the chosen zone, the tip of the needle should be inserted into the subcutaneous space. **The required technique is to do the insertion steadily, accurately, quickly and lightly to obtain the best results.**

- The Various Puncturing Methods
  - Tapping: With one hand press the eyelid of the superficial skin area. With the other hand using a needle, gently tap on the selected ocuzone about 5-7 times, taking precautions against bleeding. The needle should be perpendicular to and just touching the skin.
  - Perpendicular or Intraorbital Method: Insert adjacent to the margin of the selected ocuzone. The intraorbital needles are all perpendicular with the needle pointing toward the orbital wall. The insertion should be less than 5 mm.

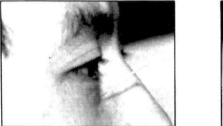
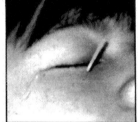

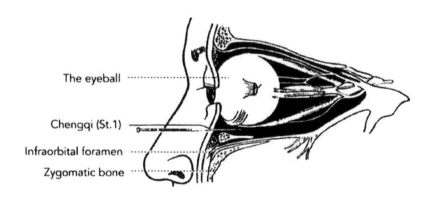

Figure 45 Perpendicular or Intraorbital Method

- Horizontal or Extraorbital Method: At the selected and well-demarcated ocuzone, insert the needle along the skin and in the appropriate direction. The insertion may go as deep, but no deeper, than the subcutaneous tissue. In a region with two ocuzones, the insertion should not cross over into the area of the adjacent zone. In the Triple Warmer regions, puncture only one ocuzone in each region. Again, the insertion should not invade the adjacent ocuzone.

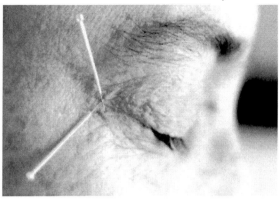

Figure 46 Horizontal or Extraorbital Method

o **Twin Needle Method:** In both perpendicular and horizontal insertions, once a needle is inserted, it is feasible to insert another needle next to it in the same direction. The therapeutic effect may thus be enhanced in this manner.

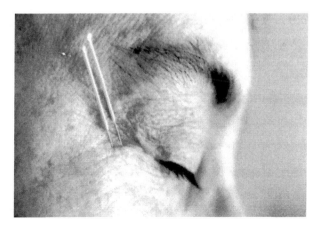

Figure 47 Twin Needle Method

o **Inner-Outer Combined Method:** At the selected periocular region, insert one needle intraorbitally and one extraorbitally. This combination will usually produce a better effect.

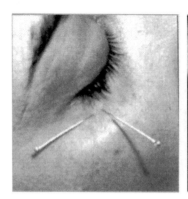 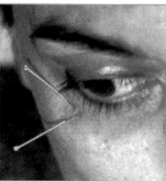

Figure 48 Inner-Outer Needle Method

Precautionary Measures

The main purpose of these precautionary measures is to avoid bleeding and swelling post-needling because the thin, soft skin of the eyelid has many capillaries inside and beneath it. Many acupuncturists had learned this technique in continuing education seminars with Hoy Ping Yee Chan, but some were still not comfortable enough to perform this technique due to fears about getting post-treatment bleeding. Dr. Chan offers the following information from her years of experience in the hope that this may relieve the tension for both practitioner and patient. Here are several situations to consider before doing periocular needling:

- **The Patient**
  o Does the patient have any fears and doubts about this method, resists the idea, or does not have confidence in the acupuncturist?
  o Is the patient emotionally unstable, especially one who has been crying before the treatment?
  o Does this patient have clotting mechanism problems such as taking anticoagulants on a long term basis, or even a senior who is taking low dose aspirin (81 mg) daily?

- Is the patient able to recline comfortably or cannot remain resting for at least 15 minutes during this treatment? This includes someone who is suffering from a serious cough or back pain. If so, you should avoid periocular needling. However, note that if the patient cannot lie on his/her back, you can also have them sit in a comfortable chair.
- If the patient is very thin, his/her eyes are deep in the orbital socket and there is not much soft tissue beneath the skin, then he/she is not a good candidate for periocular needling technique. This type of patient is more prone to bleeding following treatment and may end up with a black eye the next morning.

- **The Acupuncturist and Setting**
    - The acupuncturist should be familiar with the anatomy of blood vessels and innervations surrounding the eye and orbit.
    - New practitioners especially should practice on a pillow until comfortable enough and able to do the needling in an accurate, steady, quick and light manner.
    - The treatment room must have adequate light for the acupuncturist to perform periocular treatment; also the acupuncturist should have good enough vision to do the insertion while avoiding puncturing the small vessels on the eyelid skin that easily cause bleeding.
    - While the needle is retained during treatment, avoid applying pressure to the soft tissue surrounding the eye area. Also, the patient should refrain from chatting, coughing, sneezing or moving around, etc. As for patients suffering from partial paralysis following a stroke or one with a frozen shoulder, the affected limb can be repositioned for treatment to complete the therapy. However, under no circumstances should pressure be applied to the eye region during the needling.
    - Do not immediately send the patient off after withdrawing needles around the eye. Upon withdrawal, the acupuncturist should slightly press a sterilized piece of cotton to the skin at the point of insertion

for two to three minutes. During this time the acupuncturist can explain all the precautionary measures the patient needs to know following treatment. Finally double check that there is no bleeding before the patient leaves.

- o The patient should not engage in strenuous exercise or heavy manual work for three to four hours after treatment or, better yet, for the entire day. He/she should also be warned not to rub the eye that day since the skin of the eyelid, the thinnest part of the skin on the entire human body, is elastic and can be easily stretched. Rubbing after periocular treatment can reopen the needling area and cause renewed bleeding. The patient will show up the next day with a black eye looking like a panda.

- **Technique Alert:** To avoid bleeding, obtain *qi* upon initial insertion and no further stimulation is given. If *qi* does not arrive with the insertion of the first needle you can add in a second needle as described in the twin needle, extraocular or intraocular techniques previously described.

Dr. Chan deems that if these precautionary measures are closely observed and applied, most complications can be prevented and avoided. These tips can improve the use of this unique technique, and enhance this therapeutic effect of periocular acupuncture for the benefit of patients.

Effects, Indications and Contraindications of Periocular Acupuncture

Effects: Periocular acupuncture treats not only symptoms such as decreasing swelling, relieving pain and reducing and calming anxiety, but also treats the root of an illness by:

- Regulating the flow of *qi* and *blood*.
- Clearing and energizing the channels and collaterals.
- Eliminating stagnation.

- Harmonizing and strengthening organ function.
- Balancing *yin* and *yang*.

Indications: Periocular acupuncture can be applied as a treatment modality for any symptoms and illnesses where body acupuncture is indicated.

Contraindications:

- Patient is in critical condition, coma, mental confusion, shock or *qi* and *blood* collapse.
- Patient is trembling persistently; has involuntary restlessness.
- Patient has thickening or firm palpebrae, or has infection around the eyelid.
- Patient has a bleeding problem such as prolonged coagulation time.

Note: If you like to view or buy the book, *Window of Health---Ocular Diagnosis and Periocular Acupuncture*, please go online to Amazon.com where there are a few copies available (as of this writing) or to http://www.lulu.com/content/1385515 for the 3rd edition.

If you have more clinical questions about this technique, please contact:

Y.M Chen, Ph.D., L.Ac.
Tel: 623-551-3773;   Fax: 623-551-8912;
Address: 42104 N. Venture Dr., Ste. D 105, Anthem, AZ 85086
www.chinesehealthways.com
E-mail: chcymc@aol.com

Lee Huang, M.S., L.Ac. (Ophthalmologist in China)
Tel: 425-246-9902
Address: 2448 76th Ave SE #212, Mercer Island, WA 98040
www.ableacu.com
E-mail: lee@ableacu.com

Haipeng (Helen) J. Wong, Ph.D., L.Ac.
Tel: 425-688-0583; Fax: 425-688-0582
Address: 1106 108th Ave. NE, Suite 110, Bellevue, WA 98004
E-mail: helenwong@msn.com

APPENDIX TWO

The Most Commonly Used Chinese Herbal Formula and Its Extensive Formulas for Aging Eyes and Body

Liu Wei Di Huang Wan (Tang)
Composition:

- **Shou Di Huang (Shou Di):** Produces *essence* and enriches *blood* nourishes *yin* and moisturizes dryness. It enters into the Kidney, Liver and Heart channels.
- **Shan Yu Rou (Shan Zhu Yu):** Invigorates the liver and kidney, supplies *essence* and improves visual acuity. It enters into the Kidney and Liver channels.
- **Shan Yao (Huai Shan):** Tonifies the spleen and stomach, benefits the lung and kidney. It enters the Spleen, Lung and Kidney channels.
- **Ze Xie:** Promotes diuresis to eliminate *dampness* from the Lower Warmer and expel *heat*. It enters into the Kidney and Bladder channels.
- **Fu Ling:** Promotes diuresis to eliminate *dampness* in the Lower Warmer; strengthens spleen, harmonizes the Middle Warmer and transforms *phlegm*; calms the heart and *shen*. It enters into the Spleen, Heart, Lung and Bladder channels.

- Dan Pi (Mu Dan Pi): Clears *heat* caused by *yin* deficiency and cools the *blood*; promotes *blood* flow to remove stasis; enhances *yin* and calms the ascending liver *fire*. It enters into the Heart, Liver and Kidney channels.

Qi Ju Di Huang Wan
Liu Wei Di Huang + Qi Zi, Ju Hua

- Qi Zi (Gou Qi Zi): Nourishes *yin* and tonifies liver and kidney *yin*; benefits *blood* and *essence*; brightens the eyes. It enters into the Liver and Kidney channels.
- Ju Hua: Expels *wind* and clears *heat*; suppresses ascending liver *yang* and brightens the eyes; pacifies liver and extinguishes *wind*; clears toxins. It enters into the Lung and Liver channels.

Ming Mu Di Huang Wan
Qi Jui Di Huang + Dang Gui, Bai Shao, Ci Ji Li

- Dang Gui: Enriches *blood*, promotes blood flow and regulates menses; moisturizes dryness; loosens bowels; alleviates pain. It enters into the Heart, Liver and Spleen channels.
- Bai Shao: Nourishes *blood* and *yin*; calms liver *yang*; soothes liver *qi*; alleviates pain. It enters into the Liver and Spleen channels.
- Ci Ji Li (Ji Li): Calms liver *yang*; disperses stagnated liver *qi*; expels *wind* to alleviate pain and itching. It enters into the Liver channel.

Gui Shao Di Huang Wan
Liu Wei Di Huang + Dang Gui, Bai Shao

Zhi Bai Di Huang Wan
Liu Wei Di Huang + Zhi Mu, Huang Ba

- Zhi Mu: Clears *heat* and quells *fire*; nourishes *yin* and moisturizes *dryness*; drains Lower Warmer *heat*. It enters into the Lung, Stomach and Kidney channels.
- Huang Ba: Drains *damp heat* in the Lower Warmer and subdues kidney *fire*; clears Middle Warmer *dampness*; clears toxins. It enters into the Kidney and Bladder channels.

Jin Kui Shen Qi Wan
(Gui Fu Ba Wei Wan or Fu Gui Ba Wei Wan)
Liu Wei Di Huang + Rou Gui, Fu Zi

- Rou Gui: Warms and invigorates spleen and kidney *yang*; warms the Middle Warmer and expels *cold* to alleviate pain; promotes blood flow and generates *qi*. It enters into the Kidney, Spleen, Heart and Liver channels.
- Fu Zi (Zhi Fu Zi): Restores depleted or devastated *yang*; warms and strengthens spleen and kidney *yang*; expels *cold* and warms up the kidney *fire*; alleviates pain. It enters into the Heart, Spleen and Kidney channels.

Du Qi Wan
Liu Wei Di Huang + Wu Wei Zi

- Wu Wei Zi: Benefits *qi* and promotes the production of body fluids; contains the leakage of lung *qi* and stops coughing; restrains the *essence* and stops diarrhea; stops excess sweating; calms the *shen*. It enters into the Lung, Heart, and Kidney channels.

Mai Wei Di Huang Wan (Ba Xian Chang Shou Wan)
Liu Wei Di Huang + Mai Dong, Wu Wei Zi

- **Mai Dong (Mai Men Dong):** Nourishes *yin* and clears *heat*; moisturizes the lung and intestine, produces body fluids; nourishes the heart and clears heart *fire*. It enters into the Lung, Heart, Stomach channels.

Chai Shao Di Huang Wan
Liu Wei Di Huang + Chai Hu, Bai Shao

- **Chai Hu:** Clears external *heat* from Shaoyang channels; soothes the stagnated liver *qi*; lifts up spleen *yang* and deficiency of stomach *qi*. It enters into the Liver and Gallbladder channels.

Er Long Zao Ci Wan
Liu Wei Di Huang + Ci Shi, Chai Hu (or Wu Wei Zi)

- **Ci Shi:** Calms the liver, suppresses ascending liver *yang*, benefits *yin*; calms the *shen* and pacifies the mind; improves auditory and visual acuity; aids the kidney in grasping the *qi*. It enters into the Liver, Heart and Kidney channels. This herb is from magnetic ore.

APPENDIX THREE

Eye Exercise Chart

The eye exercise chart that follows (the full size chart can be found on the next page, 178) offers you an opportunity to give your eyes a treatment. By reading the words, you are exercising your eye muscles but this self-care exercise also allows you to rate your progress by comparing how far down the chart you can read compared to previous attempts.

1. As you read
2. this page you can
3. help exercise your eyes
4. every day by giving it a variety
5. of sizes of type to read. You can
6. read this material fast or slow while
7. it makes your eyes focus and refocus
8. and allows them to strengthen just as
9. exercise helps your body muscles to strengthen.
10. As you read you can also allow your mind to relax and
11. go easily with the flow of the words, letting the stress and
12. tension of the day dissolve into softness growing smaller and smaller
13. until there is no tension left just as the size of the type gets smaller and smaller
14. until it too dissolves into something too small to read and too small to even care about
15. because you are feeling so relaxed. By reading this exercise day after day you can continue to

1. As you read
2. this page you can
3. help exercise your eyes
4. every day by giving it a variety
5. of sizes of type to read. You can
6. read this material fast or slow while
7. it makes your eyes focus and refocus
8. and then allows them to strengthen, just as
9. exercise helps your body muscles to strengthen.
10. As you read you can also allow your mind to relax and
11. go easily with the flow of the words, letting stress and tension
12. of the day dissolve into softness growing smaller and smaller until there
13. is no tension left just as the size of the type gets smaller and smaller and then
14. dissolves into something too small to read and too small to even care about because you
15. are now feeling so relaxed. Reading this exercise day after day you can continue to improve your
16. eye health, making the muscles play even harder. Congratulate yourself now for truly helping your eyes!

Figure 49 Eye Exercise

APPENDIX FOUR

Common Eye Tests

- **Visual Acuity Tests:** The score 20/20 (V.A.) means you have normal vision at 20 feet.
  - The Pinhole Test: This test is to determine whether reduced visual acuity is due to a refractive error or to an organic vision disorder.
  - The Amsler Grid Test: This test helps to detect problems affecting the macula.
  - Color Vision Tests: This test is to check the ability to recognize color difference.
- **Perimetry:** Tests the visual field of each eye to detect patterns of vision loss that indicate specific disorders.
- **Tonometry:** Tests the intraocular pressure.
- **Fundus Fluorescein Angiography (FFA):** Shows the actual condition of vessels of the retina.
- **Gonioscopy:** Inspects the drainage angle of the eye.
- **Opthalmoscopy:** Used to evaluate any optic nerve damage and also the condition of the vessels and retina.
- **Schirmer Test:** Checks the amount of the tears produced if lower than 10 mm.
- **Optical Coherence Tomography (OCT):** Used to check and analyze the condition of the macula and retina in the diagnosis of macular degeneration.

長壽詩 — Poem of Longevity

日行九百步,	Walk nine hundred steps daily,
睡眠八小時,	Sleep eight hours every night,
飲食七分飽,	Eat only seventy percent full,
心靈常喜樂,	Be joyful in heart and soul always,
凡事要感恩.	Give thanks in all circumstances.

Author Unknown

General Index

A

A1C hemoglobin, 124
abdomen, 166
    distention and constipation, 131
acetylcholine receptors (AchR), 27
acupressure, 157
    for nose and sinus, 155
    prevention technique, 153, 154
    to benefit three hand *yin* channels, 157
Acupuncture for Stroke Rehabilitation, 114
adrenal glands and effects of alcohol, 97
adrenocorticoid hormones, 97
Age-Related Macular Degeneration. *See* ARMD
alcohol and stroke prevention, 109
amaurosis, 129
AMD. *See* ARMD
ametropia, 141
Amsler Grid Test, 77, 91, 179
anatomy, normal eye, 9
anemia, 44
anger, 99, 130, 135
angiogenesis inhibitors, 87
anterior chamber, 12, 53, 54
anterior ciliary artery, 15
anterior conjunctiva, 15
anterior eye, 11, 14
anticholinergic alkaloids, 55
anticoagulants, 171
antidepressants, 31, 98
antihistamines, 31, 98
antioxidants, 67, 76, 88
anti-VEGF therapy, 87
anti-VEGF-A therapy, 87
anxiety, calming, 170
appetite
    loss of, 32, 48, 135
    poor, 84, 129, 131, 137
aqueous humor, 12, 54, 69

ARMD, 75, 78
    acupuncture treatment, 82, 83, 85
    advanced stage, 81, 85
    causes of, 76, 81
    moxibustion, 86
    prevention and risk factors, 76, 88
    symptoms, 76, 82, 84, 85
    treatment, 51, 87
ARMD, dry form, 77, 80, 82, 85, 87
ARMD, wet form, 77, 80, 82, 87
arrhythmia, 98
arteries and veins, narrowing, 128
arteriosclerosis, 95, 96, 104, 134
 cervical, 127
    arterial and retinal changes, 103
    prevention, 109
aspirin, low dose, 169
atrophic ARMD. *See* ARMD, dry form
Atropine, 55
autoimmune disease, 27

B

Ba Zhen Tang Special Formula, 36
back and knees, soreness, 82
bagua, 4
baguo, 4
Bao Mang (Sudden Blindness). *See* CRVO, *See* CRAO, *See* diabetic retinopathy, *See* ARMD, *See* occlusion
Basic Prevention Formula, 67
BAUSCH + LOMB, 88
beating the sky-drum technique, 154
black shadows moving in front of the eye, 121
bleeding. *See also* hemorrhage
    after periocular treatment, 169, 170
    herbal treatment for, 73
    stabilized, 123
blepharitis marginalis, 31

blepharoptosis, 21, 27
    acupuncture treatment, 24
    causes of, 21
    in one eye, 23
    prevention and diet, 26
    self-massage for, 26
    symptoms of, 22
blind spot, 77
blindness, 32, 43, 45, 47, 57, 60, 78, 79, 85, 106, 117, 118
    in left field of vision of both eyes, 106
    sudden, 81, 127, 128, 129
blinks often, 33
blood, 2, 128, 133, 138
    stagnant, 15, 18, 73, 84, 128
    tonify, 26
blood and *essence*
    leaking out from the vessels, 81
    mutual growth, 81
blood glucose, 124
    herbal foot patches, 125
    high, 117, 119
blood heat, 119
blood or *cold* condition, 19
blood pressure, 7
    and alchohol use, 96
    and diabetic patient, 124
    and prescription medications, 31
    and smoking, 96
    effects of coffee, 98
    high, 65, 90, 103, 104, 109, 132, 134;
        See also hypertension
    high, during pregnancy, 104
    lowering, 97, 101
Blood Pressure Depressor machine, 113
blood stasis, 119, 128, 134
blood sugar. *See* blood glucose
blood vessels, abnormal growth, 77
Blurred Vision. See ARMD
bone marrow stem cells transplant, 87
bowel function, 67
    frequency in early morning, 89
    loose, 89, 90, 110, 131
brain, 13
    clearing, 101
    damage from smoking, 96
    infarction, 106
    retinopathy changes, 104
    visual center, 106
branch, 71, 81, 119, 130, 135
branch and root, 71
breathing, difficulty, 27
Bruch's membrane, 80
Bruno, Gene C, 87
bulbar conjunctiva, 3, 15, 50
    changes to capillary branches, 16
    colors of, 14, 19

C

caffeine and stroke prevention, 109
cancer, 128
    and B-complex warning, 65
capillary branches, color variances of, 19
Cataract Breakthrough, 65
cataracts, 45, 54, 142
    acupuncture treatment, 63
    case history, 60
    moxibustion for, 63
    supplements for, 64, 67
    surgery and ARMD link, 76
    symptoms of, 61
cataracts, congenital, 58
cataracts, diabetic, 67
cataracts, secondary, 58
cataracts, senile, 57, 74
    causes of, 58
    prognosis, 58
    progression of, 60, 61
    symptoms of, 59
    treatment, 57, 58
cataracts, traumatic, 58
central retinal artery occlusion. *See* CRAO
central retinal vein occlusion. *See* CRVO
central vision
    damage due to ARMD, 75, 78
    gradual decrease, 85
    loss of, 78, 118, 137
cerebral circulation, 102
cerebral cortex, 106

CF (counting fingers), 9, 129
channel symptoms and ocuzone selection, 165
channels and collaterals, clearing and energizing, 171
cheeks, red, 136
chelation therapy, 87
Chen Wei Li, 131
Chen Yu, 122
chest, 164, 165
   distension, 135
   oppression, 48, 84, 100, 121, 129
chest and hypochondrium
   distension, 135
   fullness, 48
chewing or swallowing difficulties, 27
cholesterol, 76, 96, 110, 128
choroid, 13, 69, 80, 81
   retinopathy changes, 104
choroidal neovascularization (CNV), 77
ciliary anterior vein, 12
ciliary body, 12
   in aging process, 141
ciliary congestion, 15
ciliary process, 12
ciliary retinal artery, 133
Classical Medical Questions, 164
Cloud Moved to Eye. See ARMD
coagulation, prolonged, 171
coffee and blood pressure, 98
cold damp, 15
cold feelings, 61
cold and blood pressure, 98
color
   difficulty discerning, 81
   vision tests, 179
Color Changed Vision. See ARMD
complexion
   dim, 120
   yellowish or blackish, 120
cones, 79, 80
confocal scanning laser ophthalmoscopy, 53
conjunctiva, 14
conjunctivitis, 16

constipation, 90, 132, 155
   and Wu Wei Zi Tea, 67
contralateral acupuncture and ocuzone selection, 167
convulsion and loss of consciousness, 104
cornea, 11, 12, 15, 22, 53, 67
   damage from rubbing, 32
   scarring, 32
   thin, 44
   ulcer, 32
coronary artery disease, 76
coronary heart disease, 127
corticosteroids, 44, 55, 58, 98
coughing, 15, 169, 175
CRAO, 128
   acupuncture treatment, 131
   positive sign for, 133
   symptoms, 129, 130, 131
   treatment, early stage, 131
CRVO, 134
   categories of, 134
   causes of, 134
   prevention of, 138
   symptoms of, 134, 135

D

damp heat, 2, 15
   middle burner, 72
damp obstruction and *phlegm*, development of, 21
dampness collects and invades the eye, 163
decongestants, 98
depression, 18, 32, 48, 129, 135
diabetes, 23, 44, 54, 58, 67, 76, 117, 118, 123, 127, 134
   and blood pressure, 98, 109
   diet for, 123
   prevention, 124
diabetes mellitus, 119
diabetic retinopathy (DR), 117, 122, 124, 125, 126
   non-proliferative form (NPDR), 117
   proliferative form (PDR), 117, 119, 120, 121

diaphragm, 164
diarrhea, 110, 131, 155, 175
   to relieve, 67
diets, 4
   and ARMD, 76
   and hypertension, 96
   and *qi* and *blood* deficiency, 71
   Chinese herbal diet formulas, 89, 90
   for blepharoptosis, 26
   for cataract treatment, 64, 65
   for diabetics, 123
   for dry eye, 39
   for preventive eye health, 152
   for stroke prevention, 109, 114
   Gou Qi Zi, 144
   Wu Zi Tea, 66
difficulty reading, writing and distinguishing faces, 77
difficulty seeing at night, 47
digestion, sluggish, 84
disorientation, 111
Distorted Vision. See ARMD
dizziness, 66, 82, 89, 100, 107, 131, 142, 147
   and eye distention, 49
   and head distension, 48
   and headache, 129
   and tinnitus, 61, 120, 130, 136
   or vertigo, 121
   unexplained, 111
Dong Mai Ying Hua. See arteriosclerosis
double vision in only one eye, 59
drainage angle, 179
dreams, many, 83
drusen deposits, 80, 81, 84
dry eye
   acupuncture treatment, 33, 34, 35, 82
   causes of, 31
   diagnosis and treatment, 32, 36
   diet for, 39
   prevention of, 40
   symptoms, 32, 33, 34, 35
Dry Eye Syndrome, 39
dryness with pain when the eyelids open and close, 34
dull and damp eyes, with fixed pupil dilation, 2
dysopsia. *See* post-stroke dysopsia
dysphoria, 130

E

ear drum vibration technique, 154
earth, 3
ECIWO, 155
edema of lower legs, 131
Eight Diagrams Theory, 4
eight diagrams, eight octants, eight regions, locations, zang-fu and 13 ocuzones chart, 163
Eight Octants Theory, 4, 159
Eight Principal Syndromes, 23
electroretinography, 133
Elschnig maculae spots, 104
embolisms, 96, 128
Embryo Containing Information Whole Organism. *See* ECIWO
emmetropia, 141
emotions
   and blood pressure, 97
   and CRAO, 128
Emperor Huangdi, 1
endarteritis, 128
endocarditis, 134
endocrine disease, 104
environment and stroke prevention, 109
ERG. *See* electroretinography
erthrocythemia, 134
essence, 2, 175
essence, qi and *blood* deficiency, 70
exercises, 57
   and blood pressure, 97
   and stroke prevention, 109
   clear blockages and move *qi*, 154
   following periocular needling, 170
   for eye care, 52, 149, 153, 177
   for prevention of presbyopia, 145
   move *qi* to eyes, 153
   to remove eye blockages, 150
   to strengthen eye muscles, 150

warming the eyes, 40
exterior conjunctiva, 16
exterior-interior relationship and ocuzone selection, 165
external rectus muscle, 146
exudates, 95, 103, 104, 118, 119, 120, 121, 137
Exudative ARMD. See ARMD, wet form
eye drops, 38, 44, 57, 65
eye examination, 52, 68, 91
    close vision testing, 9
    distance vision testing, 8
    if floaters are present, 71
    lens, 60
    location of redness, 15
    routine, 7, 46
    scheduling, 142
    with cataract, 60
eye exercise chart, 151, 177
eye orbit massage or tapping, 25, 26
eyeballs, 16, 145, 150, 165
    acupressure, 131, 132
    and ocuzones, 162
    discomfort and tension, 48
    protection, 13
    shape, 69, 147
    surface without moisture, 34
    testing pressure of, 55
    turns hard, 49
eyebrows, 13, 28
    straight, 22
    tenderness, 47
eyebrows and eyelids, skin, 22
eyelids, 13, 14, 22, 38, 166, 170
    close often, 34
    conjunctiva red and thick, 35
    finger technique to check, 28
    heavy feeling, 35
    infection, 171
    muscle weakness, 27
    swelling, 2
    sag or droop, 21, 22
    thickening, 171
eyes
    bleeding, 105
    burning sensation, 32
    color changes and ocuzones, 165
    discomfort, 47
    dry, 32
    dry, and a feeling like sand, 35
    dry eyes, mouth, pharynx and throat, 39
    dull, 33
    external, 16
    fatigued, 34
    feeling something foreign in, 32
    local disease, 70
    pressure, 135
    redness, 32
    stinging, itching, scratchiness, 32
    swelling, 134
    symptoms worse after work and when feeling tired, 49
eyesight clear and bright, 80

F

face
    expressionless, 120
    pale, 61, 120, 130, 137
    red, 99
    tidal redness, 130
falls, sudden and unexplained, 111
farsightedness. *See* hyperopia
fatigue, 15, 47, 48, 67, 71, 89, 120, 130, 137
    afternoon, 21
    and weakness, 131
    eye, 32, 83, 142
fear
    of facing into the wind, 32
    of looking at fluorescent lights, 32
    of meeting people, noise and light, 32
Fei Wen Zheng (Mosquito Flying Symptom) *See* floaters
fever, 15, 19
FFA, *See* fundus fluorescein angiography
fire, 2, 3
    excess, 15, 81
    flames upward, 72

rises up to influence the healthy eye, 2
tea for prevention of, 39
First World Conference on Acupuncture–Moxibustion, 159
five centers, burning sensation, 120, 136
five octants, 161, 162
Five Phases Theory, 3
Five Rings Theory. *See* Five Wheels Theory
Five Wheels Theory, 3, 4, 23, 80
    feng (wind), 3
    qi (energy), 3
    rou (flesh or muscle), 3
    shui (water), 3, 69
    xue (blood), 3
flashing lights in one eye, 71
floaters, 72, 73, 120
    acupuncture treatment, 74
    development of, 70
    sudden shower of, 71
    symptoms, 70
foot Taiyin Spleen channel, 81
forehead wrinkles with straight eyebrows, 22
ForeStar International, Inc, 125
fovea centralis, 13, 79
foveola. *See* fovea centralis
fu, 17, 161, 163
Fu Ren-yu, 1
Fu Yun-ke. *See* Fu Ren yu
fundus, 102
fundus fluorescein angiogram (FFA), 102, 105, 118, 133, 134, 179

G

gallbladder, 2, 15, 165
    damp heat gathering in, 72
Gao Xue Ya. See hypertension
glaucoma, 43, 52
    causes, 43
    diagnosis of, 47
    forms of, 44
    prevention key, 51
    screening methods, 52
    stages of, 44
    treatment, 51, 54
glaucoma, closed-angle, 44, 45, 54
    diagnosis, 53
glaucoma, open-angle, 44, 45, 46, 54
    acupuncture treatment, 50
    diagnosis, 48
    risk factors, 44
    symptoms, 46-49
    treatment, 48
glaucoma, secondary, 45, 133, 138
forms of, 54
    causes of, 55
    neovascular, 54
gonioscopy, 53, 179
gout and blood pressure, 98

H

Haiping (Helen) J. Wong, 172
hair analysis, 64
He Gu Cui Technique, 28, 29
head, 166, 167
    heavy, 100
    heavy with vertigo, 129
headache, 135, 142
    frontal, 47, 155
    heavy, 101
    sudden severe, 111
    with dizziness, 99
heart, 2, 3, 15, 103, 104, 167
    and coffee, 98
    and smoking, 96
    irritation, 135
    palpitations, 131, 137
    retinopathy changes, 104
heart and spleen, dual deficiency, 137
heart *qi* deficiency, 128
heart *yin*, to nourish, 67
heat, 2, 67, 84, 122
    developing disorder, 19
    excess, 15, 37
in the five hearts, 100
heat-fire, 67
Hei Feng Nei Zhang, 45

Heidelberg Retinal Tomography, 53
hemianopia, 106
hemorrhage, 106, 121, 123, 134
    and acupuncture treatment, 137
    in vitreous humor, 118
    retinal, 118, 119, 133, 135, 137
    small dot, 118
    subconjunctival, 15
    vitreous, 138
hemorrhagic spots, 119, 120
herbal diets
    for *qi* and *blood* dual deficiency, 90
    tonify liver and kidney, 89
    tonify spleen and boost *qi*, 89
    tonify spleen and kidney, 89
herbal honey tea, 52
herbal patches, *See* patches
HM (hand motion), 60, 129
Hoy Ping Yee Chan, 60, 145, 159, 168, 170
HRT. *See* Heidelberg Retinal Tomography
Hua Tuo, 1
Huang Feng Nei Zhang, 44, 45
Huangdi Nei Jing, 1
hunger and eats frequently, 119
hyaluronic acid, 69
hyperlipemia, 125
hyperlipidemia, 134
hyperopia, 76, 141
hypertension, 44, 127, 131, 138, *See* also blood pressure, high
    arterial and retinal changes, 103
    complications of, 104
    in diabetes, 125
    prevention, 109
    primary, 95, 104
    risk factors, 95
secondary, 98
    symptoms, 99, 100, 101
    treatment for, 104
hypertensive retinopathy, 102, 103, 104, 132
    neuroretinopathy, 104
    symptoms, 99
hyperthyroidism and blood pressure, 98

I

I-Cap, 67
implantable miniature telescopes, 87
impotence and polyuria at night, 120
inability to focus on nearby objects, 12
inability to recognize and interpret visual stimuli such as faces, words, 106
increasing need for more light when reading or doing close work, 59
infarction, 54
infection, 15, 134
    eye, 21
    outer eye, 122
    parasitic, 18
inferior oblique muscle, 146
inferior rectus muscle, 146
injury
    eye, 15, 21, 23, 44, 58, 70
    face, 15
inner and outer canthus, 3
insomnia, 49
International Congress of Chinese Medicine & Acupuncture, 145
intraocular lens (IOL) implant, 58
intraocular pressure (IOP), 46, 51, 55
    effects of medication, 55
    high, 43, 44, 47, 54, 55, 128
    low, 47, 50
    measurement of, 52
    normal reading, 46
    rising, 45, 54
    testing, 179
intraorbital method, 166
involuntary restlessness, 171
iris, 3, 11, 12, 15, 53
irisitis, 15
irritable, 48
ischemia, 118
itching, alleviate, 67

J

Jian Fei (Useless Eyelid). *See* blepharoptosis
Jin Ming, 67
Jing Jing (Vitreolent Eye Drops), 65

John Hopkins Medical Center, 114

K

Keith-Wagener-Barker classification, 103
Kemeny, Stuart, 65
keratitis sicca, 15, 32. *See* also dry eye
kidney, 2, 3, 69, 80, 81, 103, 104
    and alcohol use, 97
    house of *water* and *fire*, 80
    internal *cold* or *wind*, 15
    relationship to the macula, 80
    relationship to the pupil, 80
    retinopathy changes, 104
    weakness and ARMD, 80
    yin and *yang* balance, 80
kidney disease, 104
    and blood pressure, 98
kidney *essence*
    benefit, 67
    deficiency, 21
kidney *qi*, 2
    and *yin* and *yang* balance, 66
    deficiency, 58
Kondrot, Edward C, 87

L

lacrimal apparatus, 11
lacrimal glands, 31
Lanzhou College of TCM, 145
Lao Shi (Old Eye's Vision). *See* presbyopia
laser photocoagulation, 87
lateral geniculate body, 106
Lee Huang, 171
lei huo jiu (moxa stick), 63
lens, 12, 54
    aging process, 57, 58, 141
    cloudy areas, 59
leukemia, 134
levator palpebrae muscle, 14
Li Pin Qing, 85
Li Rui, 67
Liaoning College of Traditional Chinese Medicine, 4, 159
light perception, *See* LP

light reaction. *See* LR
limbs
    dusky purple color at tips, 121
    sore and tight, 131
    weak, 27
Ling Shu (*Miraculous Pivot*), 1
lipids, 96, 125
lips, dusky purple color, 121
lips, throat, mouth, dry but no desire to drink, 136
liver, 3, 15, 69, 80, 81, 165
    and alcohol use, 97
    and cataract development, 66
    and eye, 1
    and protein conversion, 96
    point of entry, 81
    soup, 39
liver-gallbladder *fire* flaming upward, 135
liver *qi*
    blocked, 72
    deficiency, 58
    stagnation, 81, 129
liver *wind* internal stirring upwards, 130
liver *yang*, hyperactive, 72
liver *yin*, deficiency, 81
liver-kidney
    and lung *yin*, deficiency, 39
    essence, *qi* and *blood* deficiency, 61
    imbalance and vitreous disease, 69
    qi deficiency, 70, 72, 81
    yin deficiency, 88, 110, 128
    yin, tonify, 144
loss of coordination, 107
loss of interest for doing activities, 32
low back and knees
    sore with weakness, 61, 89, 136
    tiredness, 120
    weakness, 119
Lower Blood Pressure Neck Patch, 101, 110
Lower Warmer, 162, 164, 165, 173, 175
LP (light perception), 9, 60
LR (light reaction), 9, 11, 60, 129
Lu Feng Nei Zhang, 44, 45
Lui Hui Ying, 64

lung *qi*
    symptoms of collapse, 2
    tonify, 26
lungs, 2, 3, 15, 165
luo mai, 2, 21, 23, 108, 131, 136, 153

M

MacuCare, 88
macula, 13, 75, 76, 79, 80, 81, 118, 133, 179
    and foot Taiyin Spleen channel, 81
    blood or fluid under, 77, 83
    cherry red spot, 133
    edema, 118, 120, 137
    relationship to the pupil, 80
    relationship with organs, 80
macular degeneration. *See* ARMD
malnutrition, 71
massage. *See* self-massage
medial rectus muscle, 146
memory loss, 111
Meniere's Disease, 67
mental confusion, 171
meridians
    12 regular, 2
    arm, 157
    Bladder, 2, 153, 155, 162, 173, 175
    extra channels, 2
    Gallbladder, 2, 153, 154, 164, 176
    Governing Vessel, 2, 153, 155
    Heart, 2, 162, 173, 174, 175, 176
    Kidney, 2, 157, 162, 173, 174, 175, 176
    Large Intestine, 2, 162
    leg, 157
    Liver, 2, 81, 157, 162, 173, 174, 175, 176
    Lung, 2, 162, 173, 174, 175
    muscle channels, 2
    Pericardium, 2, 157
    relationship with the eyes, 2
    Ren Mai (Conception Vessel), 2
    Small Intestine, 2, 154, 162
    Spleen, 2, 157, 162, 173, 174, 175, 176
    Stomach, 2, 162, 174, 175

    three foot *yang*, 2
    three foot *yin*, 2
    three hand *yang*, 2, 157
    three hand *yin*, 2, 157
    Triple Warmer, 2, 154, 157
    yang Linking, 2
    yin linking, 2
metal, 3
microaneurysms, 117, 118, 119
microcurrent therapy, 87
Middle Warmer, 162, 164, 165, 175
mind
    and high blood pressure, 97
    foggy, 48, 83
Ming Dynasty, 1
Miraculous Pivot, 164
Mosquito Flying Symptom. See floaters
mouth
    and throat, dryness, 34, 100
    bitter, 48, 130
    bitter and dry, 48, 135
    dry, 32, 49, 83, 119
    sticky phlegm and bitter taste, 129
moxibustion, 25
    for ARMD, 83, 86
    for blepharoptosis, 26
    for cataract treatment, 63
    for treatment of glaucoma, 51
    herbal string, 112
    pen, 112
    walnut shell glasses, 86
muscles
    fatigue easily if doing repetitions, 27
    weakness, 27
myasthenia, 21, 27
    acupuncture treatment, 28
    difference from blepharoptosis, 27
    differential diagnosis and treatment, 28
myopia, 44, 141, 145

N

naming eye diseases, difficulties, 4
National Eye Institute, 43, 87
nausea, 100, 142, 147, 150

and vomiting, 104
nearsightedness. *See* myopia
nebula, removing, 67
muscle tension, 155
needling, periocular, 166
    horizontal, 167
    inner-outer combined, 168
    perpendicular, 166
    precautions, 168
    tapping, 166
    twin needle, 167
neovascular ARMD. *See* ARMD, wet form
neovascular glaucoma, 54
nervous personality
    and high blood pressure, 97
night driving problems, 60
night sweats, 83
nocturia, 89
noise and blood pressure, 97
non-neovascular ARMD, 77
non-steroidal anti-inflammatories, 98
normal vision. *See* emmetropia
nose, throat and mouth dryness, 33
NPDR. *See* diabetic retinopathy
numbness, 107
    in the limbs, 121
    of the face, arm or leg, 111
Nutrition, Health and Disease, 64

O

Observation of Changing Conditions of the Whole Body, 16
occipital area, 106, 109, 154
occlusion, 117, 118
    medical exams for, 133
    phlegm obstruction, 121
    phlegm-stasis, 121
    retinal vein, 104, 133, 137
    static *blood*, 121
ocular diagnosis and periocular acupuncture, 4, 159, 165
Oculax Acupoint Patch, 38, 63, 88
oculomotor nerve, paralysis, 23
Ocuvite, 67, 88
ocuzones, 17, 24, 160, 161, 162, 165, 166
    and needling, 167
    capillary changes in, 25
    finding locations of, 159
    Heart (Zone 9), 33, 34, 131
    Kidney (Zone 3), 34, 35, 82, 123, 131, 143
    Liver (Zone 6), 33, 34, 82, 123, 131, 143
    Lower Warmer (Zone 13), 50, 85, 123, 143, 144
    Lung (Zone 1), 34, 35
    Middle Warmer (Zone 8), 50, 83, 85, 123, 144
    principles of therapeutic selection, 165
    Spleen (Zone 11), 25, 35, 83, 123
    Upper Warmer (Zone 5), 25, 33, 34, 35, 50, 82, 83, 85, 123, 131, 143, 144
OD, 8
Ophthalmology Hospital of the Chinese Medicine Research Academy, 131
opthalmoscopy, 52, 179
optic disc, 46
    and CRAO changes, 133
    red color with unclear edge and hemorrhages, 137
    retinopathy changes, 104
    swelling, 104
optic nerve, 13, 43, 106, 133
    damage, 43, 47, 52, 55
    damage evaluation, 179
    destroyed, 47
    imaging, 53
    increased cupping, 44
orbicularis oculi muscle, 14
orbiculus ciliaris. *See* pars plana
orbit, 14, 131, 150, 169
orbital pressure, high, 128
orbital septum, 14
orbital socket, 169
orbital wall, 166
organ function, harmonize and strengthen, 171
original essence, 80
OS, 8
OU, 8

overweight, 100, 121
   and blood pressure, 97
oxidative damage and diabetic cataract, 67
oxygen therapy, 132

P

pain
   and tension in the eyes and head, 48
   back, 169
   eye, 36, 47
   in the shoulder, elbow and wrist, 112
   joint, 32
   relieving, 170
palms, hot, 49
palpebrae. *See* eyelids
palpebral conjunctiva, 14
palpebral internal artery, 16
palpebral margin, 14
palpitations, 48
pancreas, 125, 126, 165
paralysis, 111
   left limbs, 106
   partial, following a stroke, 169
Parkinson's, prescription medications, 31
pars plana, 12
patches, 38, 88, 101
   hot eye, 152
   lower glucose, 125
   lower blood pressure, 101, 110
   Oculax, 33, 63, 88
pelvic cavity, 165
Peng Jingshan, 4, 16, 159, 164, 164
perimetry, 179
periocular acupuncture
   and acupuncturist, 169
   and patient, 169
   contraindications, 169, 171
   effects of, 170
   indications, 171
   needling technique, 165, 166
   post treatment bleeding, 170
   precautionary measures, 170
   treatment room, 169
peripheral vision, 78
   loss of, 43, 47
periphlebitis, 134
perspiration, spontaneous, 120
phacoemulsification, 57, 58
phlegm and *dampness*, 21, 119
phlegm heat rises upwards, 128, 129
phlegm with nausea, 48
photodynamic therapy, 87
pian, 111
pinhole test, 179
Poem of Longevity, 180
point injection, 132
polyuria, 120
posterior pole, 118
post-menopausal syndrome and blood pressure, 98
post-needling bleeding and swelling, 168
post-stroke dysopsia, 95, 106
   acupuncture treatment, 108
   causes, 106
   prevention, 109
   symptoms, 106
presbyopia, 12, 141, 145
   categories, 141
   differential diagnosis and treatment, 142
   prevention, 142, 145
   symptoms of, 141, 142
prescription medications, 31, 40, 55, 57, 87, 132
   and blood pressure, 98
   and embolism, 128
   blood thinning, 52
   side effects, 109
preventive methods
   early stage eye disease, 4
   general eye care, 149
   self-care techniques, 153
Project ORBIS International, 57
Prostigmin, 27
pseudoexfoliation syndrome, 54
ptosis. *See* blepharoptosis
pulse
   deep and rough, 84
   deep and weak, 61, 120

empty and weak, 120, 137
fine, 34, 49, 71, 82
fine and deep, 119
fine and rapid, 33, 135, 136
rough and deep, 131
slow and weak, 85
string-like, 48, 130
  and rapid, 99, 100, 135
  and rough, 121, 129, 135
  and slippery, 84, 100, 121, 129
  and tight or rough, 101
slippery and rapid, 48
weak, 83
weak, pauses at regular intervals, 130
wiry and fine, 48
pupil, 3, 9, 11, 12, 15, 17, 44, 52, 60, 138
and locating ocuzones, 160
color changes in glaucoma, 45, 47
dilated, 45, 49, 129
dilating for exam, 15, 118
relationship to the kidney, 80
red color, 72
pupil light reflex, 11

Q

qi, 2
disorders *of*, 135
failure to arrive, 170
move, 126, 155, 157
obtaining, 28
weakness of, 19, 130
qi and *blood*, 1, 2
abnormal raising, 128
balance, 153
collapse, 171
dual deficiency, 71, 72
increase flow of, 155
move, 101, 154
move to eyes, 38, 43, 50, 52, 63, 123, 150
regulate, 51, 171
stagnation, 19, 129, 135
qi and *yin*
deficiency of root, 119

deficiency patterns, 32
dual deficiency, 119, 120
qi deficiency, 119
and *blood* stasis, 130
with palpitations, 135
qi stagnation and *blood* stasis of branch, 119
Qian Diagram, 159
Qin Feng (Wind Invaded). *See* blepharoptosis
Qing Feng Nei Zhang (Indigo Wind Internal Obstruction), 44, 45, 46, 47
Qing Guang Yan (Indigo Light Eye). *See* glaucoma

R

rainbow-like circles around light sources seen, 47, 49
reflex constriction, 137
refractive error, 179
retina, 12, 13, 69, 79, 80, 81, 103, 133, 135, 141, 145, 149
and blood pressure, 98
and floaters, 69
and sudden blindness, 132
atrophy or degeneration, 137
bleeding, 135
'blood bank of', 80
changes in CRVO, 134
changes in diabetic retinopathy, 117
complications of cataract surgery, 58
detached, 13, 71, 104, 117, 118, 121
edema, 132, 137
evaluating damage of, 179
hemorrhage, 104, 118, 119
hemorrhage and swelling, 95, 137
hypertensive changes, 99, 103
swelling, 104, 118, 120, 121
white fibers, 118
retinal arteries, 95, 103, 137
CRAO changes, 133
hypertension changes, 103
occlusion, 127, 128
thrombosis, 128

retinal pigment epithelium (RPE), 80
retinal vein, 118
    occlusion, 137
retinal vessels, new growth, 121
rods and cones, 13, 79
root, 54, 71, 81, 119, 130, 170
RPE. *See* retinal pigment epithelium
rubbing eyes too often, 32

S

salt water eye bath, 38, 152
Sanjiao. *See* Triple Warmer
scanning laser polarimetry (GDx), 53
Schirmer Test, 31, 179
Schlemm Canal, 12
sclera, 12, 13, 15
sclerosis, 128
sea of blood, 81
second heart of the body point, 157
Second Hospital Affiliated with Tianjing College of TCM, 108
seeing bright colors as dull, 59
self-massage, 4, 26, 91
    eye, 52, 64, 88
    eyes and ears, 64
    for eye prevention, 155
sense organs, 165
Shang Bao Xia Chui (Upper Eyelid Dropped Down). *See* blepharoptosis
shen, 7
shen gao (god's gel). *See* vitreous humor
Shen Shi Yao Han, 1
Shen Shui Jiang Ke (Tears Almost Dried Out). *See* dry eye
Shi Wang Mo Bing Bian (Retinal Diseases), 95
Shi Wu Bian Xing (Distorted Vision). *See* ARMD
Shi Zhan Hun Miao (Blurred Vision as Mist). *See* CRVO, *See* diabetic retinopathy, *See* ARMD, *See* vitreous humor

Shi Zhan You Se (Blurred Vision as Seen Color in the Eye). *See* ARMD, *See* vitreous humor
shock, 44, 171
shortness of breath, 71, 120
Six Excessive of Atmospheric Influences, 23
six-channel pattern identification system, 81
Sjogren Syndrome. *See* dry eye syndrome
sleep, 67
    disturbed, 48
sleeplessness, 15, 21, 32, 99, 135
    with dreams, 82, 130
slit lamp-microscope, 60
SMD. *See* ARMD
smoking, 76, 90, 96
    and hyperlipemia, 125
    and hypertension, 125
    and stroke prevention, 109
Snellen Chart, 7, 8, 9
source *qi*, 2
speech, garbled, slurred, trouble understanding, 107, 111
    loss of, 111
spleen, 2, 3, 15, 80, 81, 165
    and liver and kidney *qi*, *yin* and *yang*
    and kidney, dual deficiency, 120
    balance and vitreous health, 74
spleen *qi*, 2
    and *yin* and *yang* balance, 66
    deficiency, 21, 58
    deficiency and blurred vision, 81
    fails to move *damp* and transform *phlegm*, 21
    sinking, 81
spleen *yang*
    disturbed, 72
    tonify, 26
stagnation
    arterial, 128
    dampness, *phlegm* and *blood*, 81
    eliminating, 171

Standard Formula, 122
static blood spots, 121
steaming the eyes, 152
Steenblock, David A, 87
stereo nerve photographs, 53
sticky mucous around the eyelashes in the morning, 32
stomach, 2, 165
stool, thin and sloppy, 137
stress, 18, 32
    and CRAO, 128
    and stroke prevention, 109
stroke, 23, 106
    occipital lobe, 106
    only attacking the eye, 108
    prevention, 101, 109
    self-test, 112
    supplements for, 114
    warning signs, 107
strong spirit and brightness in the eyes, 2
Su Wen (Plain Questions), 1
Sudden Blindness. See ARMD
sudden blindness, prevention, 132
Sun Si-miao, 1
superior oblique muscle, 146
supplements
    for ARMD, 87
    for stroke, 114
    specific for eye health, 67
sweating, excessive, 175
swelling, reducing, 170
sympathetic nervous system, 97
syndrome differentiation and ocuzone selection, 165

T

talk, does not like to, 130
tang formula, 72, 87
tarsus, inflammation of, 31
taste, bitter, 48, 90, 99
tear film evaporation, 31
tear production, measurement, 179
tearing, 32
teas, for diabetics, 124
thirst, 84, 119
three foot *yang*, 158
three foot *yin*, 157, 158
throat dry, 120
thromboembolism. *See* embolism
thrombosis, 128
TIA. *See* trans ischemic attack
tinnitus, 49, 66, 82, 89, 99, 100
tiredness of low back and knees, 120
Todd, Gary P, 64, 67
tong shen. See pupils
tongue
    crimson with slight yellow coat, 49
    damp purple with static spots, 101
    dim red with stasis speckles, 84
    dusky purple with static spots, 121
    faded red with purple static spots and thin white coat, 135
    pale, 61, 137
    purple, 129
    red, 35, 99
    swollen, 120
    swollen and pale with white coating, 120
    with greasy coat, 100
    with purple spots, 130, 131
    with thin coating, 85
    with white coating, 83
    with dry coat, 33
    without a coat, 34
    with thin coating, 82, 83, 119, 136
    with thin, dry yellow coat, 100
    with yellow coat, 48, 99, 130, 135
    with yellow greasy coat, 48, 84, 129
tongue and lips pale, 71
tonometry, 52, 179
too lazy to speak, 137
too tired to talk, 120
trabecular meshwork, 12
transient ischemic attack (TIA), 111
    self-test, 112
trembling, 171
triglycerides, 90, 110

Triple Warmer, 167
   and eye, 163
   disease location and ocuzones, 165
   theory of ocular acupuncture, 163
   treatment boundaries, 165
trouble talking, 111
Tufts' USDA Human Nutrition Research Center on Aging, 58
tunnel vision, 47, 49, 133

U

ultraviolet light, 58, 65, 76, 91, 153
unsteadiness, unexplained, 111
upper extremities, 164, 165
Upper Warmer, 162, 164, 165
upset, 48, 99
urination, frequent, 67
urine, large volume especially at night, 61

V

vasospasm, 128
vertigo, 67
vision
   blurred, 47, 49, 60, 61, 77, 81, 99, 100, 118, 119, 120
   clearing, 101
   dim spot in front of eyes, 82
   dimming, 107, 111
   distorted or disturbed, 48, 77, 84
   fuzzy or hazy, 59
   partial, 121
   poor or weak, 121, 131, 149
   varies, 32
vision loss, 49, 55, 84, 95, 107, 111, 117, 126, 135
   and distortion, 82, 83
   detecting patterns of, 179
   gradual, 99
   in CRVO, 134
   partial, 108
   rapid decreases accompanied by headache, 104
   severe, 81, 119, 127
   slow, 101
   sudden, 80, 129, 130
   temporary, 136
   when looking at a bright scene or background, 60
visual acuity, 7, 60, 176
   loss of, 32, 106
   reduced to CF or HM, 129
   tests for, 179
visual field, 133
   blind spot in center of, 77
   destroyed, 47
   narrows (tunnel vision), 49
   partial blockage, 71
   test, 52, 179
Vitreolent Eye Drops, 65
vitreous body, 69, 121
vitreous chamber, 12
   blood in, 72, 74, 138
vitreous humor, 12, 69, 74, 104, 135
   degeneration of, 70
disease symptoms, 71, 72
   function of, 69
   hemorrhage, 118, 119, 138
   white fibers, 118
voluntary muscle, weakness, 27

W

walnut shell moxibustion glasses, 86
wan formula, 72, 87, 111
Wang Kentang, 1
Wang Ming Fong, 81
Warring States Period, 1
water, 2, 3, 163
   insufficiency, 81
weakness, 15, 82, 107
   general, 32, 71, 83, 85, 90
   lower back and knees, 119
   sudden, 111
Wei Zheng. See myasthenia
wind heat, 36
wind invasion, prevention of, 26
wind, phlegm, fire, and stasis four aspects, 99
wind-phlegm, 21

Window of Health---Ocular Diagnosis and Periocular Acupuncture, 159, 171
wood, 3
Wu Danyi, 123
Wǔ Feng Nei Zhang (Five Kinds of Wind Cause Internal Obstruction). *See* glaucoma
Wū Feng Nei Zhang, 45, 54
Wu Zi Tea, 66

X

Xiao Ke. See diabetes mellitus
Xiao Ke Mu Bing (Eye Diseases from the Thirsting and Wasting Disease). *See* diabetic retinopathy
Xinming, extra point, 51, 85

Y

Y. M. Chen, 171
Yan Ke Da Quan (A Complete work of Ophthalmology). see Shen Shi Yao Han
Yan Zhong Feng (Eye Stroke), 95, *See* post-stroke dysopsia
yang
   eye relationship, 159
   hyperactivity, 128
yang qi, 1
   prevented from rising, 21
   raise up, 153
yin
   enrich, 126
   eye relationship, 160
   sinking, 88, 124

yin and *blood,* deficiency, 119
yin and *yang*
   balance, 40, 80, 88, 91, 110, 124, 153, 171
   balance, in liver, kidney, spleen and heart in CRVO, 138
yin and *yang* of *blood,* balance, 157
yin deficiency, 15, 36, 40, 123
   and dry *heat*, 119
   causing hyperactive *fire*, 136
   in post-menopausal women, 25
Yin Hai Jing Wei (Essentials of Ophthalmology), 1
yuan qi, 163
Yuan Yi Nei Zhang (Round and Nebulous Internal Obstruction). *See* senile cataract
Yun Mu Yi Jing (Cloud and Fog Move into the Eye). *See* diabetic retinopathy, *See* vitreous humor

Z

zang-fu, 1, 2, 3, 4, 71, 161
Zhang Wei Rong, 138
Zhang Wencai, 111
Zhang Yulian, 108
Zheng Zhi Zhun Sheng (Guidelines in Syndrome Differentiation and Treatment), 1
zhi wei bing, 4
Zhu Zhong Dong Qi (*Qi* Is Moving Inside the Eye). *See* vitreous humor

Formula Index

Formula 1: Bu Zhong Yi Qi Tang---Codonopsis & Astralagus Combination, 23, 28, 62, 83

Formula 2: Ren Shen Yang Tong (Ying) Tang---Ginseng & Rehmannia Combination, 23

Formula 3: Zheng Rong Tang---Reforming Face Formula, 24

Formula 4: Fu Gui Li Zhong Tang---Aconite, Ginseng & Ginger Combination, 28

Formula 5: Xiao Yao San---Dang Gui & Bupleurum Combination Powder, 33

Formula 6: Sheng Mai San---Engender Pulse Powder, 33, 120

Formula 7: Sang Bai Pi Tang---Mulberry Bark Formula, 33

Formula 8: Qi Ju Di Huang Wan---Lycium, Chrysanthemum & Rehmannia Formula, 34, 50, 62, 143

Formula 9: Zeng Ye Tang---Increase Liquid Formula, 35

Formula 10: Chu Shi Tang---Clear Dampness Formula, 35

Formula 11: Ba Zhen Tang---Angelica & Ginseng Eight Combination, 36, 72, 130, 144

Formula 12: Gan Mai Da Zao Tang---Licorice & Jujube Combination, 40

Formula 13: San Zi Yi Ming Tang---Three Seeds Beneficial Vision Soup, 40

Formula 14: Dan Zhi Xiao Yao San---Moutan + Gardenia + Dang Gui & Buplerum Formula, 48

Formula 15: Ling Yang Jiao Tang---Antelope Horn Formula, 48

Formula 16: Huang Lian Wen Dan Tang---Coptis Hoelen & Bamboo Combination, 49

Formula 17: E jiao Ji Zi Huang Tang---Donkey Hide with Hen Egg Yolk Formula, 49

Formula 18: Shen Qi Tang (Fu Gui Di Huang Tang)---Aconite, Cinnamon + Rehmannia Six Formula, 50, 120

Formula 19: Qing Guang Ming Shi Tang---Clear Vision Brighten the Eyes, 52

Formula 20: Shi Hu Ye Guang Wan---Dendrobium Combination, 62

Formula 21: You Gui Wan---Eucommia & Rehmannia Formula, 62

Formula 22: Yi Yin Shen Qi Wan---benefit the Kidney Yin and Qi Pill + Zhen Zhu Mu (Pearl Powder), 63

Formula 23: Man Jing Zi Powders + Pork, 64

Formula 24: Xie Zhu Ming Mu Ye---Musk and Pearl Eyedrops, 65

Formula 25: ZYM Di Yan Ye, 65

Formula 26: Liu Wei Di Huang Wan---Rehmannia Six Formula, 66, 110, 120

Formula 27: Bu Shen Wan (Tu Si Zi Wan)---Cuscutae Semen Pill, 66

Formula 28: Wu Zi Tea---Five Seed Tea, 66

Formula 29: Ming Mu Di Huang Wan---Rehmannia Eye Bright Pills, 71

Formula 30: Shi Quan Da Bu Wan---Ginseng and Angelica Ten Combination Pill, 72

Formula 31: Wen Dan Tang---Bamboo & Hoelen Combination, 72, 121

Formula 32: Ling Xue Tang---Staunch the Bleeding Combination, 73
Formula 33: Tao Hong Si Wu Tang---Persica and Carthamus Four Herb Combination, 73, 132, 136
Formula 34: Er Chen Tang---Citrus & Pinellia Combination, 73, 84
Formula 35: Si Wu Tang + Wu Zi Wan---Angelica Four and Five Seed Combination, 82, 119
Formula 36: Zhi Bai Di Huang Tang---Anemarrhena, Phellodendron & Rehmannia Formula, 84, 100, 136
Formula 37: San Ren Tang---Triple Nut Combination, 84
Formula 38: Xue Fu Zhu Yu Tang---Persica & Cartharmus Combination, 84, 101, 121
Formula 39: Tian Ma Gou Teng Yin---Gastrodia & Uncaria Combination, 99, 130
Formula 40: Ban Xia Bai Zhu Tian Ma Tang---Pinellia & Gastrodia Combination, 100, 111
Formula 41: Er Zhi Wan---Ligustrum & Eclipta Combination, 100
Formula 42: Tian Ma Gou Teng Pian---Gastrodia & Unicaria Tablet, 101
Formula 43: Bu Yang Huan Wu Tang---Astragalus and Chinese Peony Combination, 108, 130, 131, 136
Formula 44: Jiang Dan Gu Chun Pian---Crataegi Citrus Fruit Tablet, 108
Formula 45: Zuo Gui Yin---Restore Left Kidney Decoction, 66
Formula 46: Standard Tonification Formula, 122
Formula 47: Tong Qiao Huo Xue Tang---Clear Orifice and Quicken Blood Formula, 129
Formula 48: Di Tan Tang---Rinse Phlegm Formula, 129
Formula 49: Da Ding Geng Zhu---Settle Down the Wind Formula, 130
Formula 50: Long Dan Xie Gan Tang---Gentiana Combination, 135
Formula 51: Chai Hu Shu Gan Tang---Bupleurum & Cyprus Combination, 135
Formula 52: Gui Pi Tang---Angelica, Ginseng & Longan Combination, 137
Formula 53: Di Zhi Wan, 142

Differential Diagnosis Index

Ascendant Liver *Yang* Transforming into *Wind*, 99

Blood Stasis, 131

Deficiency and Weakness of Spleen *Qi*, 62

Deficiency is More of Liver-Kidney *Yin*, 62

Deficiency is More of *Qi Essence*, 62

Deficiency of *Blood* and Liver *Fire* Flames Upward, 63

Deficiency of *Qi* and *Blood*, 23

Dual Deficiency of Heart and Spleen, 137

Dual Deficiency of Liver and Kidney *Yin*, 143

Dual Deficiency of *Qi* and *Yin*, 120

Dual Deficiency of Spleen and Kidney, 120

Fluid and Tear Shortage, 34

Heat attacks Kidney causing Kidney *Yin* Deficiency, 142

Kidney *Yang* Deficiency, 62

Liver and Kidney *Yin* Deficiency, 60

Liver *Fire* Flaming Upward, Frenetic Movement of *Hot Blood*, 72

Liver *Heat* Engender *Wind*, 48, 50

Liver *Qi* Depression and Liver *Yin* Deficiency, 32

Liver *Qi* Stagnation Transform *Fire*, 48, 50

Liver *Wind* Internal Stirring Upward, 130

Liver-Gallbladder *Fire* Flaming Upward, 135

Liver-Kidney Deficiency, 82

Liver-Kidney Deficiency and *Fire* Flaming Upward, 100

Liver-Kidney Dual Deficiency, 49, 51

Liver-kidney *Essence, Qi* and *Blood* Deficiency, 61

Liver-Kidney *Yin* Deficiency, 34, 71

Yin Deficiency *Wind* Stirring, 49, 50

Treatment Principles Index

A
aid the kidney in grasping the *qi*, 176
alleviate pain, 174, 175

B
benefit *blood* and *essence*, 174
benefit eyesight, help conjunctivitis, 67
benefit hearing by moving blockages in all the associated acupuncture points, 154
benefit *qi* and promote the production of body fluid, 175
benefit *yin*, calm the *shen* and pacify the mind, 176
boost *qi* and nourish *yin*, 33
boost *qi* and quicken *blood*, 130
boost *qi* and stop chronic hemorrhage, 137
brighten the eyes, 174

C
calm liver and extinguish the *wind*, 130
calm liver *wind*; clear the *heat*, 101
calm liver *yang*, 67, 99, 174
calm liver, suppress ascending liver *yang*, 176
calm the mind and aid sleep, 154
calm the heart and *shen*, 173
calm the *shen*, 175
clear and drain liver *fire*, 135
clear *blood* stasis, bleeding more than three months, newly formed vessels and scars, 122
clear external *heat* from Shaoyang channels, 176
clear *heat* and act as diuretic, 67
clear *heat* and quell *fire*, 174
clear *heat* caused by *yin* deficiency and cool the *blood*, 174
clear *heat*, cool down *fire*, 48
clear *heat*, cool the *blood*, 99
clear *heat* first, then tonify kidney *yin*, 142
clear *heat*, promote diuresis, and clear eyesight, 66
clear *heat* to brighten the eye, 84, 152
clear liver fire and anger, 99
clear liver *heat* and extinguish *wind*, 48
clear liver *heat* and transform *phlegm*, 49
clear liver *heat*, enrich *yin*, 52
clear liver *heat-fire*, 67
clear lung *heat* and nourish lung *yin*, 33
clear the eyesight, 65
clear the *luo mai*
 and move *blood*, 153
 and brighten the eye, 121, 130
 and open the orifices, 130
clear Middle Warmer *dampness*, 175
clear toxins, 174, 175
contain the leakage of lung *qi* and stop coughing, 175
control *wind* and expel *phlegm*, 24
cool and stanch the bleeding, 73, 84, 136
cool *blood* and transform stasis, 119

D
deficiency of liver-kidney *yin* and *blood*, 50
disinhibit *water* and clear the eye, 84
dispel *dampness* and clear the *heat*, 72
dispel *dampness* and expel *phlegm*, 84
dispel stasis and clear the network vessels, 100, 108, 131
dispel *wind* and boost *qi* to nourish *blood*, 23
dispel *wind* and release pain, 100
disperse stagnant liver *qi*, 174
drain damp *heat* in the Lower Warmer and quell kidney *fire*, 175
drain Lower Warmer *heat.*, 174

dry the *dampness* and expel *phlegm*, 121

E

enhance *yin* and calm ascending liver *fire*, 174
enrich and nourish liver and kidney *yin*, 34, 62, 143
enrich and harmonize *blood*, 176
enrich *blood*, 174
enrich *blood* to brighten the eye, 63
enrich liver and kidney function, 72
enrich *qi* and nourish *yin*, 120
enrich *yin* and bring down *fire*, 63, 84, 100, 136
enrich *yin* and moisten the *dryness*, 119
enrich *yin* and nourish *blood*, 49
expel *cold* and warm up kidney *fire*, 175
expel *phlegm* and clear the vessels, 129
expel *wind-heat* on the eye and head, 67, 174
expel *wind* to alleviate pain and itching, 174

F

for headache - to dispel *wind*, release pain, 100
for hyperactivity of *yang*, 130
for white exudate on the retina, clear liver *fire*, disinhibit *water*, 99
fortify and boost spleen *yang*, 62
fresh bleeding, 122
fresh hemorrhage on the retina, 135

H

harmonize the stomach and expel *phlegm*, 100, 111
harmonize the stomach to calm down, 49

I

improve auditory and visual acuity, 176
increase *blood* flow to the eyes and clear the vessels., 152

invigorate the liver and kidney, supply *essence* and improve visual acuity, 173

L

lift up spleen *yang* and deficiency of stomach *qi*, 176
liver *wind* internal stirring upwards, 130
liver-kidney dual deficiency, 51

M

moisten and enrich fluid, 119
moisturize dryness and move bowels, 174, 176
moisturize the lung and intestine, produce body fluids, 175
move *qi*, quicken *blood* and clear network vessels, 101
move *qi* and tonify the *blood*, 85
move *qi* and relieve depression, 135

N

nourish *blood* and restrain *yin*, 174
nourish heart and clear heart *fire*, 175
nourish liver and moisten the eyes, 40
nourish *yin* and clear *heat*, 175
nourish *yin* and engender liquid, 35
nourish *yin* and moisturize dryness, 174
nourish *yin* and tonify liver and kidney *yin*, 174

P

pacify liver and extinguish *wind*, 174
produce *essence*, enrich *blood*, nourish *yin* and moisturize dryness, 173
produce fluids, 35
promote blood flow and generate *qi*, 175
promote *blood* flow and regulate menses, 174, 176
promote *blood* flow to remove stasis, 174
promote diuresis to eliminate *dampness* in the Lower Warmer and expel *heat*, 173
promote eyesight and preserve kidney *essence*, 67

Q

qi and *blood* dual deficiency, 90
quicken *blood,* dispel stasis, 24, 73, 84, 121, 132, 136
quicken *blood,* dissipate *phlegm,* 100
quicken *blood,* open orifices, 129
quicken *blood,* transform the proliferative membrane, 121
quicken *blood* flow, clear the vessels, 24
quicken *blood* flow, dilate the arteries and dispell stagnation, 132

R

relieve headache of *cold* and *wind-heat* type, 67
restore depleted or devastated *yang,* 175
restrain the *essence* and stop diarrhea, 175

S

soften hardness and expel *phlegm,* 84
soften liver and extinguish *wind,* 49
soothe liver *qi,* 174, 176
soothe liver and nourish *blood,* 33
stop excess sweating, 175
strengthen spleen, harmonize the Middle Warmer and transform *phlegm,* 173
supplement both *qi* and *blood,* 72
supplement liver and kidney *yin* and dispell stasis, 82
supplement liver and kidney *yin,* cool the *blood* and stop bleeding, 100
support and nourish heart and spleen, 137
support *blood* and stanch blood flow, 137
support nutrition and brighten the eye, 64
suppress ascending liver *yang* and brighten the eyes, 174
suppress liver *yang* and clear liver *fire heat,* 67
suppress liver *yang* and clear vision, 90

T

tonification, 122
tonify and benefit liver and kidney, 62, 101
tonify and supplement kidney *yang,* 62
tonify *blood,* 26
tonify heart *yin,* nourish *blood* and calm the *shen,* 40
tonify kidney and warm up the whole body, 157
tonify kidney *yang,* 66, 67
tonify kidney *yang* and *essence,* 50
tonify kidney *yin, yang* and *blood,* 66
tonify liver and kidney, 66, 89
tonify liver and kidney *qi,* 67
tonify liver and kidney *yin,* 66, 71, 110
tonify *qi* and *blood* in liver and kidney, 50
tonify *qi* and *blood,* harmonize *yin* and *yang,* 36, 144
tonify *qi* and liver function, 67
tonify *qi* and quicken *blood,* 131
tonify *qi* and quicken *blood,* dispel stasis and clear the *luo,* 108
tonify spleen and boost *qi,* 89
tonify spleen and inhibit the *dampness,* 35
tonify spleen and kidney, 89
tonify spleen and kidney *yang,* 28
tonify spleen and stomach, benefit the lung and kidney, 173
tonify spleen *qi,* 26, 67
tonify spleen *yang,* 28
tonify spleen *yang* and *qi,* 23, 83
tonify *yin, yang* and *blood,* 66
transform *phlegm* and resolve depression, 121
transform turbidity and dissolve fat, 108

W

warm *yang* and boost *qi,* enrich kidney and act an astringent, 120
warm and invigorate spleen and kidney *yang,* 175
warm the Middle Warmer and expel *cold* to alleviate pain, 175

About the Authors

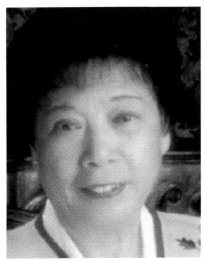

Hoy Ping Yee Chan, O.M.D.

Hoy Ping Yee Chan, OMD, holds the national board certification as Diplomate of both Acupuncture and Chinese Herbology, Retired, NCCAOM. She was one of the first independent acupuncture practitioners in Washington State after the bill legalizing acupuncture was passed in 1985. Dr. Chan holds a doctoral degree in Oriental Medicine from SAMRA University in Los Angeles, U.S.A. and, before immigrating to America, had graduated from Beijing (Peking) Medical University in China. There she practiced Western medicine for 18 years, sometimes combining it with traditional Chinese medicine.

Within the last thirty years, Dr. Chan has shared her theories, medical knowledge, clinical experience and health care recommendations in acupuncture schools, continuing education seminars, television, newspaper interviews, public communities, and made presentations at acupuncture conferences worldwide.

In 1996, Dr. Chan compiled the first edition of *Window of Health---Ocular Diagnosis and Periocular Acupuncture,* published by Northwest Institute of Acupuncture and Oriental Medicine. She was one of the first few acupuncturists in the United States to learn this unique advanced microacupuncture technique and tried her best to spread it across the nation.

In 2006, the first issue of *Acupuncture for Stroke Rehabilitation* was published by Blue Poppy Press. Dr. Chan was the chief compiler on the selections of three decades of information from numerous acupuncture and Chinese medical magazines. This is the first book about acupuncture for stroke written in English and contains information about how Chinese medicine understands stroke, clinical acupuncture treatments for stroke rehabilitation, various special acupuncture techniques to treat specific post-stroke symptoms, opinions from Western medical researchers on acupuncture treatments and stroke prevention information.

In 2007, the World Journal of Acupuncture-Moxibustion, Beijing, China published a special issue of the book *Acupuncture in the Whole World* (針行天下). In it, Hoy Ping Yee Chan was selected as one of the world's outstanding acupuncturists. This was a great honor to her.

Although Dr. Chan has retired from clinical practice, she drew her energy to write this new book, *Chinese Medicine for Aging Eyes*. She hopes this book will continue to be a way to share her experience and knowledge of acupuncture and herbal treatments with younger practitioners for the benefit of their patients, by providing practitioners with the advanced material about common eye diseases of seniors beyond what they were taught in school. She wishes more acupuncturists had expanded knowledge to take care of elders who are suffering vision damage so that these seniors will have a better life in their old age.

Dr. Chan also especially hopes that there will soon be better integration between practitioners of traditional Chinese and Western medicine to bring about improved treatment of eye diseases commonly found in seniors.

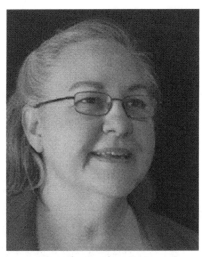

Carole Conlon, L.Ac.

Carole Conlon, M.T. (ASCP), L.Ac., holds the NCCAOM national board certification as Diplomate of Acupuncture. Following a 1984 graduation from the Northwest Institute of Acupuncture and Oriental Medicine in Seattle and an internship at the Chongqing Institute of Traditional Chinese Medicine in Chongqing, China, she worked as an acupuncturist in Washington State for 21 years, eventually specializing in Nogier's Auriculomedicine method and a focus on clearing the emotional aspects of disease. Prior to her acupuncture studies, Carole worked as a registered medical technologist in a variety of hospital settings for 12 years, including five years serving in Barrow and Bethel Alaska Indian Health Service Hospitals.

Now residing in New Mexico, Carole continues to work with patients through needle-free ear acupuncture, energy work and, lately, is studying and providing nutritional counseling to help patients improve their basic core health. In addition, Carole has been drawn to writing and publishing in order to reach out to more people to help them improve their own health and wellbeing.

During the time Carole practiced traditional acupuncture, she also began developing a pendulum testing and healing method called *LifeWeaving*. Then in 2006, a paradigm-shifting course revealed her life destiny and, in order to better embrace that mission, Carole began to upgrade and transform both herself and the pendulum work, and began working more on an energetic, emotional and spiritual approach with patients.

Today, Carole's healing and teaching methods are directed to helping people restore their ayni—their sacred relationship—with themselves, with each other, with their environment, with their own health, and even with existence itself through auricular acupuncture, nutritional counseling, LifeWeaving Clearing, teaching and writing.

On a personal note, Carole enjoys the abundant sunshine of New Mexico and very much likes dragons.

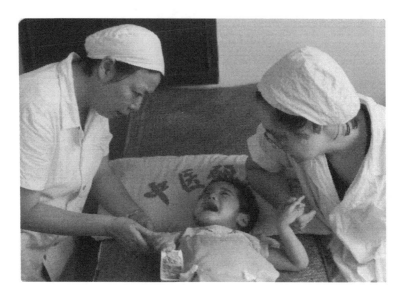

Hoy Ping Yee Chan (L) and Carol Conlon (R) working on a young patient in Chongqing, China in 1984

Other Books Available from the Authors

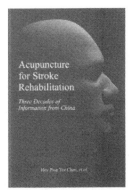

Acupuncture for Stroke Rehabilitation---Three Decades of Information from China
by Hoy Ping Yee Chan, O.M.D., et.al.

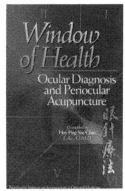

Window of Health---Ocular Diagnosis and Periocular Acupuncture
Compiled by Hoy Ping Yee Chan, O.M.D.

- This book provides a comprehensive look at cerebral vascular accident (stroke) including
- Understanding stroke diagnosis and treatment both in Western and traditional Chinese medicine
- Review of standard acupuncture therapy for stroke based on TCM differential diagnosis
- Acupuncture treatments for post-stroke symptoms
- Clinical trials and examples of special techniques used by Chinese medical stroke experts
- Stroke Prevention

PRODUCT DETAILS:
 ISBN: 1-891845-35-7
 AUTHOR: Hoy Ping Yee Chan
 176 pages, Soft Cover
 Available from www.bluepoppy.com (or call 800-487-9296) and www.Amazon.com

The first edition was published by Northwest Institute of Acupuncture and Oriental Medicine in 1996. This book is a compilation of Professor Peng Jingshan's work and his book, *Ocular Needle Therapy* (眼針療法), including observation of the eye for diagnosis and periocular needling technique.

Note that the third edition of this book includes extra information on iridology, compiled by Ralph Wilson, N.D., L.Ac.

PRODUCT DETAILS:
 First Edition: ISBN: 0962266523
 AUTHOR: Hoy Ping Yee Chan
 5 1/2 X 8 1/2
 85 pages, Soft Cover
 Available from www.Amazon.com

 Third Edition: ISBN: 9780962266522
 AUTHOR: Hoy Ping Yee Chan
 Published Dec. 9, 2007
 8 1/2 x 11
 116 pages, Soft Cover
 Available at
 www.lulu.com/content/1385515

LifeWeaving Clearing Manuals and Laminated Charts
by Carole Conlon

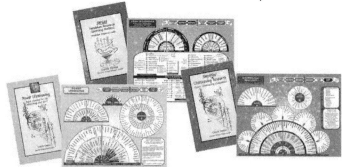

Power LifeWeaving---Rapid Clearing for the Mind, Body and Spirit
Simplified LifeWeaving Research---Power LifeWeaving Companion
PRSM Pendulum Research Sourcing Method---Pendulum Diagnosis

Using these LifeWeaving dowsing charts can help to restore ayni by letting you identify and quickly eliminate many energy blocks between you and your surroundings, or that stop you from healing. The companion manuals give a complete overview of the LifeWeaving System and describe all elements found on the charts, basic and advanced protocols, and energy healing tips.

The Tiny Ayni book series:

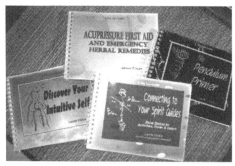

- *Acupressure First Aid and Emergency Herbal Remedies*
- *The Pendulum Primer*
- *Connecting to Your Spirit Guides*
- *Discover Your Intuitive Self*

These coil-bound, soft cover books are 5 1/4" x 4 1/4" and range from 29 - 56 b&w pages. These books offer a complete mini-version of each topic. Detailed information on each book is available at www.AyniWritePress.com.

Please visit www.AyniWritePress.com for more information on these books and be sure to fill out the contact form to be advised of future titles by these authors.

Made in the USA
San Bernardino, CA
06 June 2016